THE FUTURE OF PSYCHOLOGICAL THERAPY

The psychotherapy and counselling profession has recently experienced far-reaching changes because of the development of evidence-based medicine and managed care systems. *The Future of Psychological Therapy* brings together leading counsellors, psychotherapists, psychological therapists and managers to address how these changes are beginning to affect all aspects of the psychotherapy and counselling profession. It evaluates the impact of these developments, shows how they affect practitioners' capacity to care, anticipates future developments and offers a coherent and viable approach to research and practice.

The book draws on psychotherapeutic theory to develop insight into managed care and engages in qualitative microphenomena research into the complexities of clinical practice drawing on cutting edge developments. It aims to establish a balanced counselling and psychotherapy profession by:

* opening up a debate about these far-reaching developments which threaten the profession;
* challenging the rhetoric of accountability, audit, transparency and measurement of care;
* exposing the danger of sleeping through these momentous changes in the counselling and psychotherapy profession.

The Future of Psychological Therapy is a timely and important book, examining the psychotherapy profession's approach to managed care and evidence-based research, and discussing whether a balanced, coherent and viable counselling and psychotherapy research and practice culture can be established. It will be of interest to practitioners, academics and policy makers in the field, non-clinical professionals and anyone who is interested in psychological therapy and addressing the worldwide deterioration in psychological health.

John Lees is Senior Lecturer in Mental Health at the University of Leeds and counselling and psychotherapy practitioner in private practice in London and Sussex. He is editor of a Routledge journal, *Psychodynamic Counselling* (now *Psychodynamic Practice*), a Routledge book series, co-editor of four books and has published numerous book chapters and professional articles. He designed an MSc in Therapeutic Counselling, was programme leader of that course for twelve years and co-designed three other therapy-orientated postgraduate courses at the University of Greenwich. He has spoken at conferences in the United States, Japan and Australia, has been visiting scholar at colleges or universities in Japan, Australia and India, and has designed a course on anthroposophic psychotherapy in Japan.

'Incisive and timely, this collection of critiques of contemporary professional therapy contains astute analysis and radical political challenge regarding the neoliberal trend of managed care, IAPT and associated societal dynamics, presented by some of the most knowledgeable observers in the field. It is a gauntlet of a book, not to be missed by all who care about the future of mental health and psychological therapies.'

– Colin Feltham, Emeritus Professor of Critical Counselling Studies, Sheffield Hallam University

'The helping professions have been increasingly influenced by the prevailing political and economic climate since the 1980s. This book contains a set of timely reflections on how counselling and psychotherapy are affected by the current zeitgeist. They make it abundantly clear that the modernist paradigm, as exemplified by both a state-endorsed version of "therapy" such as IAPT and NICE's over-emphasis on the value of randomised controlled trials, is totally incompatible with non-prescriptive, potentially transformative, "authentic" therapy. This book is an important wake-up call to the pernicious effect of various aspects of neoliberalism, particularly the practices and language associated with it. In the Brave New World of "managed care", public discourse is in danger of falling into a moral vacuum, leading to a general loss of the real meaning of "care". I hope that this book will be widely read.'

– Dr Els van Ooijen, psychotherapist, counsellor and supervisor in private practice; Visiting Lecturer in Consultative Supervision to the University of South Wales

THE FUTURE OF PSYCHOLOGICAL THERAPY

From managed care to transformational practice

Edited by John Lees

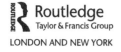

Routledge
Taylor & Francis Group

LONDON AND NEW YORK

First published 2016
by Routledge
2 Park Square, Milton Park, Abingdon, Oxon OX14 4RN

and by Routledge
711 Third Avenue, New York, NY 10017

Routledge is an imprint of the Taylor & Francis Group, an informa business

British Library Cataloguing in Publication Data
A catalogue record for this book is available from the British Library

Library of Congress Cataloging in Publication Data
The future of psychological therapy : from managed care to transformational
  practice / edited by John Lees.
    p. ; cm.
  Includes bibliographical references.
  I. Lees, John, 1951– , editor. [DNLM: 1. Psychotherapy—trends—Great
  Britain. 2. Managed Care Programs—Great Britain. 3. Mental Health
  Services—Great Britain. 4. Psychotherapy—manpower—Great Britain.
  5. Quality of Health Care—Great Britain. WM 420]
  RC489.R43362.19689'14—dc232015032879

ISBN: 978-1-138-88639-1 (hbk)
ISBN: 978-1-138-88638-4 (pbk)
ISBN: 978-1-315-70829-4 (ebk)

Typeset in Bembo and Stone Sans
by Florence Production Ltd, Stoodleigh, Devon, UK

CONTENTS

CONTRIBUTORS

The late **William Bento, PhD**, was a licensed transpersonal clinical psychologist at Folsom State Prison Crisis Treatment Centre in Folsom, CA. He was also adult educator and supervisor of mental health at Camphill Soltane in Glenmore, PA, former Associate Academic Dean at Rudolf Steiner College, Fair Oaks, CA, psychotherapist in private practice and Executive Director of the Anthroposophic Psychology Associates of North America conducting certificate programs in Anthroposophic Counseling Psychology in four regions in the United States. He authored numerous articles on psychology, new star wisdom, education and cultural commentary, *Lifting the Veil of Mental Illness* (2004), *Psycho-diagnostic Approach to Personality Disorders: An Understanding of Personality through Spatial Orientation* (2009), and was co-author of *The Counselor: As if Soul and Spirit Matter* (2015).

Richard House, PhD, is a trained humanistic counsellor/psychotherapist, a chartered psychologist (BPS), and a trained Steiner teacher. Formerly Senior Lecturer in Psychotherapy and Counselling at the University of Roehampton (2005–12), he latterly lectured in Early Childhood at the University of Winchester (2012–14). Now a freelance educational consultant, he is a founder-member of the Alliance for Counselling and Psychotherapy and of the Independent Practitioners Network (IPN). The co-editor of *Self and Society: International Journal for Humanistic Psychology*, his published books include *Therapy Beyond Modernity* (Karnac, 2003), *In, Against and Beyond Therapy* (PCCS Books, 2010) and *Against and For CBT* (PCCS Books, 2008; co-edited with Del Loewenthal). Richard has been writing and campaigning against the statutory regulation and over-mechanisation of Britain's 'psy' field since the early 1990s.

John Lees, PhD, is Senior Lecturer in Mental Health at the University of Leeds, counselling and psychotherapy practitioner in private practice in London and Sussex, and founder editor of a Routledge journal, *Psychodynamic Counselling* (now *Psychodynamic Practice*). He has edited a Routledge book series, co-edited four books and published numerous book chapters and 44 professional articles, 19 of which have been peer reviewed. He has designed an MSc in Therapeutic Counselling, was Programme leader of that course for 12 years and co-designed three other therapy-orientated postgraduate courses, at the University of Greenwich. He has spoken at academic/professional conferences in the United States, Japan, and Australia, has been visiting scholar at colleges and universities in Japan, Australia and India and has designed a course on anthroposophic psychotherapy in Japan. For further details see http://johnleestherapy.com/.

Del Loewenthal is Professor of Psychotherapy and Counselling, and Director of the Research Centre for Therapeutic Education at the University of Roehampton, where he also convenes Doctoral programmes. Del is also a Visiting Professor at the University of Athens, in the Department of Philosophy, Pedagogy and Psychology. He is an existential-analytic psychotherapist, chartered psychologist and photographer and is founding editor of the *European Journal of Psychotherapy and Counselling*. He is chair of the Universities Psychotherapy and Counselling Association and former founding chair of the UK Council for Psychotherapy Research committee. Del also has small private practices in Wimbledon and Brighton. His most recent publications include: *Post-existentialism and the Psychological Therapies: Towards a Therapy without Foundations* (2011), *Phototherapy and Therapeutic Photography in a Digital Age* (2013), (with Andrew Samuels) *Relational Psychotherapy, Psychoanalysis and Counselling: Appraisals and Reappraisals* (2014) and *Critical Psychotherapy, Psychoanalysis and Counselling: Implications for Practice* (2015). He is currently writing *Existential Psychotherapy and Counselling after Postmodernism*.

Stuart Morgan-Ayrs, BA, BSc, MSc, DHy, trained in psychoanalysis, clinical hypnotherapy and stress management counselling from 1993–1996 with ASM. Post qualification Stuart has completed extensive CPD training in a wide range of areas including an MSc in Psychology. He currently works out of Edinburgh, with additional clinics across central Scotland. He is a Fellow of the Royal Scottish Society of Arts, the Royal Society of Public Health, the Institute of Health Promotion and Education and an associate fellow of the Royal Society of Medicine. He is subject to voluntary regulation as a hypnotherapist via the CNHC, and is listed on both the CNHC and FHT AR accredited voluntary registers.

John Nuttall is Head of School of Psychotherapy and Psychology and Professor of Integrative Psychotherapy and Research Methods at Regents University London. He is a professional psychotherapist in private practice, has had a long career in senior management in industry and commerce, and is a Certified Management Consultant and Chartered Marketer. John has written widely on management and psychotherapy and his special interests include psychotherapy integration, organisation theory, and the provision of counselling and psychotherapy in the community. He is also honorary psychotherapist and Chair of the charity West London Centre for Counselling, a major provider of therapeutic counselling in primary care.

Rosemary Rizq, PhD, is a Chartered Psychologist, a Senior Practitioner member of the British Psychological Society's Register of Psychologists Specialising in Psychotherapy and a UKCP-registered psychoanalytic psychotherapist. She is currently Principal Lecturer in Counselling Psychology at Roehampton University and until 2013 worked for many years as Specialist Lead for Research and Development for an NHS Primary Care Service. She now has a private practice in West London. Rosemary was submissions editor for Psychodynamic Practice from 2004–2010 and has published widely in the field of organisational dynamics and psychotherapeutic practice and training. She has recently authored several papers exploring unconscious organisational dynamics within IAPT services.

Andrew Samuels was chair of the UK Council for Psychotherapy and co-founder of both Psychotherapists and Counsellors for Social Responsibility and of the Alliance for Counselling and Psychotherapy. He co-founded the journal *Psychotherapy and Politics International*. He trained as a Jungian analyst and his pluralistic clinical approach blends post-Jungian, relational psychoanalytic and humanistic elements. He is Professor of Analytical Psychology at Essex and holds visiting professorships at New York, Goldsmiths, Roehampton and Macau Universities. His many books have been translated into 19 languages and include *The Plural Psyche* (1989), *The Political Psyche* (1993), *Politics on the Couch* (2001), *Relational Psychotherapy, Psychoanalysis and Counselling* (edited with Del Loewenthal, 2014), *Persons, Passions, Psychotherapy, Politics* (2014) and *A New Therapy for Politics?* (2015). His rants on many topics, including the state of the therapy world, are at www.andrewsamuels.com.

Ian Simpson was Head of Psychotherapy Services at a major London teaching hospital for 20 years. He retired from the NHS four years ago and continues to have a small private practice offering individual and group psychotherapy, supervision and reflective practice for staff teams. He has written about issues of containment and group dynamics in 'Containing the Uncontainable; A role for staff support groups' in *Psychological Groupwork with Acute Psychiatric Inpatients (2010)*, and CAT in groups (with Norma Maple), in *Cognitive Analytic Therapy: Developments in Theory and Practice (1995)*, and about contextual safety within the NHS. 'We all know about "Good Enough" but Is it "Safe Enough?"', in *Group Analysis (1995)*.

Nick Totton is a body psychotherapist, trainer and supervisor in private practice. He is author or contributing editor of 14 books, including *Psychotherapy and Politics* (Sage), *Body Psychotherapy: An Introduction* (Open University Press), *Wild Therapy: Undomesticating Inner and Outer Worlds* (PCCS Books) and *Not A Tame Lion: Writings* *on Therapy in its Social and Political Contexts* (PCCS Books), as well as many chapters, papers and articles. He is consulting editor (previously editor) of Psychotherapy and Politics International, and current chair of Psychotherapists and Counsellors for Social Responsibility.

Jay Watts is a Clinical Psychologist and Psychotherapist. She is Honorary Senior Research Fellow at Queen Mary College, University of London, as well as being in full time private practice. Until 2012, she was Psychology Lead and Research Lead in one of the two NHS boroughs where IAPT was initially piloted, managing the knock on effects on dramatically increased secondary care referrals in a local community unparalleled in its cultural diversity and poverty. Jay has also led an Early Intervention in Psychosis Team, developed critical psychology courses as Senior Lecturer in Psychology at City University, and supervised multiple individuals and groups working in IAPT. She is Practice Editor for the European Journal for Counselling and Psychotherapy, and has published widely.

FOREWORD

Andrew Samuels

'We shall fight them on the beaches.' It turned out not to be necessary then, but for many therapists this is how it feels now. Like Britons in 1940, they fear the worst. Such therapists already feel in their bones that they have lost what I call 'the battle for the soul'.

In the United States and Britain, with resonances in other Western countries, a battle has broken out regarding emotional distress (and 'illness'): How we talk about it, whether we try to measure it or not, and – crucially – what we do about it. Behind this battle for ownership of the soul lies contemporary culture's profound ambivalence regarding psychotherapy and counselling. Many countries have now opted for what they believe to be a quick and effective form of therapy, Cognitive Behaviour Therapy (CBT) which, proponents say, has been scientifically measured to have proven effects in relation to sufferers of anxiety and depression. Hence, in the UK, well-established approaches, such as humanistic, integrative, family systemic and psychodynamic are vanishing from the NHS. Either CBT or a watered down version of it that I call 'state therapy' gets the funding.

A high proportion of psychotherapists and counsellors feel that, whatever their many satisfactions in the work with clients and patients, they have failed in their generative task of securing and extending into the future the practices and values of that which they profess. They feel they have lost the battle for the soul.

This book is a gift for them.

Yet such a collection begs the question: Who are the opponents of these often polemical chapters? Where are the baddies – the cynical politicians, the self-promoting academics, the leading lights in those schools of therapy that are getting the money? So – who and what did the authors have in mind as they wrote? Heraclitus said that *Polemos* (meaning strife) was 'the father of all, the kind of all'. Yet for many therapists, trained to value reflection over action, balance over passion, and keeping one's head down over potentially self-revealing political action, polemic is strange territory.

A polemical work in this field – and, if you think about it, in this field there are only polemical works, created with an opponent in mind – will excite equally polemical responses. Unpleasant as it may be sometimes, it is probably better than being ignored. I found this when, on 27 October 2007, in a letter to the *Guardian*, I was one of the first to challenge the seemingly obvious benevolence of the Improving Access to Psychological Therapies scheme. I wrote that IAPT would offer 'second class therapy for citizens deemed to be second class', and the blasts I received were many and mighty. (You can read the letter at the end of this Foreword; the entire ensuing exchange with a leading CBT practitioner, and chair of the professional organisation who were the beneficiaries of the creation of the IAPT scheme, may be found in Veale and Samuels, 2009, pp. 41–56.)

With the polemical *opposition* to the book in mind, I decided in my Foreword to raise and critically discuss a number of questions arising from reading the chapters. 'Be thou my enemy for friendship's sake' wrote Blake – and I write in that spirit though I am not in any way an enemy of the viewpoints expressed herein, and have stood shoulder to shoulder with the majority of contributors for many years. Yet if you really want to be a pluralist in this or another field you have to buy into a process of incorrigible bargaining, competition and negotiation. I noticed that only a very few of our authors did anticipate what might be said against their ideas, but the majority did not.

Here we go with the questions.

Aren't you people self-interested, pursuing professional (and hence material and reputational) advancement?

When I was chair of UKCP, we struggled to counter the point that our opposition to closures of NHS psychotherapy services, then to be replaced by IAPT centres, was merely a last throw of an embattled group of elitist professionals who had had it all their way for far too long. Indeed, some of what we were defending had deformed over time into something rather difficult to defend. For example, in some areas of the country, the privileging of psychodynamic and psychoanalytic ideas meant that our efforts to protect services had to be done with, as they say, a clothes peg on the nose.

I think it is very hard to separate concern for self from concern for other, especially when, for most therapists, their work is definitely a job (denied, often) as well as a vocation (shared with pride, always). Hence, when the discourse is of what will benefit the client or society, the shadow dimension needs to be held in mind. What we found in UKCP was that our opponents could accept that the rhetoric of client choice and client benefit was not incompatible with idealistic people seeking to practice a healing art in the way that they had been trained to do it. Moreover, when the values that underpinned even traditional psychotherapy and counselling were picked out – as opposed to doomsday scenaria about 'mental health' epidemics if therapy services were cut – the flavour of the argument changed.

It did not mean that opponents of psychodynamics-dominated services rolled over, but they seemed more receptive to the other side.

Why are you therapists so left-wing?

The question does not only refer to the authors in this book. I have heard this so many times – in Westminster and Whitehall, in therapy circles that feel silenced, and from clients – and never quite know how to reply. It is probably the case that, these days, the majority of therapists are critical of the political, economic and social *status quo* – in their private lives. But in their work settings, or at conferences on attachment or neuroscience, the kinds of critiques of capitalism and neo-liberalism that you can read herein do not get uttered by the majority. The therapists who do speak out are often highly libertarian/anarchist and/or profoundly idealistic in a humanistic and/or spiritual vein. Many have had a radical past in the 1960s and 1970s and 'Thatcherism' is still a live issue for them. Of course, it *is* a live issue, and it *should be* a live issue, but this is probably not where the plumb line in contemporary Britain falls (NB this was written before the result of the 2015 General Election was known).

You see, those who extol IAPTs, and see nothing wrong in the way NICE controls what is and is not acceptable research methodology, have somehow managed to convince everyone that they are *not* ideologically driven. This is something that many of this book's authors take on and they brilliantly reveal the theorising and the sets of assumptions that drive what is happening in the therapy world in our time. Yet the problem remains – and it is a problem for the left generally – that we are seen as more out of touch than our colleagues whose views tend in a rightwards direction.

One thing that has perplexed me since reading the book for the purpose of writing its Foreword is the stress in some chapters on what can seem like limitless freedom in the practice of psychotherapy and counselling. This is rarely qualified yet we all know that such oceanic freedom does not exist. In my view, there is no possibility of free association in any meaningful sense in the therapy world today. The state, the society, and training with its stress on containment, boundary and safety – all of these operate in the therapist's mind.

That is why we need a book like this and the kind of campaign it can be part of. We are all constrained, and not just by the human condition. I understand the main thrust of the book to be that the nature of the dominant contemporary constraints is what is being challenged, and no claim for absolute freedom is being made. In other words, we understand that there will always be chains but dispute that the current ones are the only ones there could be. This is not to devalue Utopic thinking which I see as absolutely necessary in the first instance for any kind of transformational change, whether personal or social.

Aren't you truly out of touch if you can't see the benefits of IAPT?

The paid staff at UKCP could not see why the psychotherapist members would not welcome more citizens getting more therapeutic help than ever before. Yes, people like me said all the obvious things to them about quality versus quantity and referred to people wanting to have a relationship with their therapist. Similarly, one of the academics who was in at the founding of the IAPT scheme spoke at a conference of IAPT as a 'socialist endeavour'. He later resigned because he became aware that IAPTs were cooking the books to return more favourable results than was in fact the case.

I think that what some of us refer to as 'state therapy', which is still mostly what IAPTs offer, needs to be distinguished from 'real' CBT (to the extent that there is a discrete therapy called CBT). This may mean, for some, including me, being more generous towards CBT than is their natural inclination. Otherwise, progressive, radical and critical therapists end up seeming to be against practically everything.

Who are you fooling when you praise the 'therapy relationship' to the skies?

Let me explain what this question is about. All the writers in this book have positive things to say about the creation and co-creation of the therapy relationship (and, implicitly, the therapeutic alliance). 'It's the relationship, stupid!' But isn't it time to question this as the litmus test of the kinds of therapies that escape the neo-liberal IAPT pit? For example, we know now how critical the role of the client is in the therapy process (see Norcross, 2011). Movement and exploration depend more on where the client is in their trajectory of change than on the quality of the therapy relationship.

I have been doing research on what therapists offer in terms of the therapy relationship by carrying out a systematic scanning of the blurbs on therapists' websites, which use a combination of a soft sell, purple prose, and overblown claims and promises. Reading this disgustingly wonderful stuff leads me to muse that it might not be a bad thing if the relentless 'me-me-me' in terms of the therapist's presence were to be reduced a bit.

There may be an analogous problem with the idea of the therapeutic alliance. So important is this idea that at least one modality college of the UKCP requires applicants to write an essay on it. (Incidentally, when this college wanted to call itself the college of 'relational psychotherapy', all the other colleges protested that (a) they were relational too, and (b) it would give the relational college an unfair commercial advantage.)

Viewed from an egalitarian perspective, the therapeutic alliance involves a claim that the therapist is always ready, willing and able to embark on the therapy, offering an invitation to the client to join the alliance – and now the client has to climb up to the therapist's level. The therapist contracts to assist the client in coming up to the therapist's level. The therapist is there, above the flood waters of hate and ambivalence, now the client has to scramble up and join her. Don't therapists know that failures to achieve the therapeutic alliance are often as much to do with the blind spots and wounds of the therapist as much as they are of the client? Or that many clients never really enter anything resembling an alliance, but still do useful, though unblessed, work?

Finally, the relentlessness with which the value added by the therapy relationship is promoted considers therapy within a value-free and hermetically sealed container. The ways in which the diverse political positions of the therapist and the client, together with myriad social, cultural, economic and ecological factors, impact on the therapeutic alliance and the therapy relationship do not receive sufficient attention. The one-size fits all approach to therapy seems to me to be alive and kicking (maybe to differing degrees) on both sides of the battle for the soul.

Isn't there a contradiction between rejecting any research at all into therapy as inappropriate on the one hand and critiquing NICE on the other hand?

Some therapists reject any commitment to or investment in research into therapy. They say that it is not the kind of activity that can be researched, and that each therapy encounter is so unique that there are no overarching patterns that a researcher could discern without doing violence to the phenomenon.

Others believe that what is holding back a fairer and more client-friendly disposition of therapy in the country is the blinkered approach of NICE to what constitutes appropriate methodology. Succinctly, although its documents allow for non-RCT research evidence to be considered, in practice NICE does not recognise any other kind of research methodology. This is of huge significance. Psychotherapy, it has been said, is one of the most researched human enterprises that has ever existed. Yet only a few tiny bits of the research opus pass muster at NICE – and this is mainly because they have been tailor-made to get past the assessment committees. (And let's not forget that the backgrounds of those who populate those committees is by no means representative of the field as a whole. It is actually a major and scandalous stitch-up.)

But does it matter, that's the question, and the book does not offer a uniform answer. If psychotherapy cannot be researched, then what is the point of arguing for a wider range of existing (and maybe new) research to be considered by NICE?

There is also the 'if you can't beat them join them' approach to be considered. Should we not do RCTs of our own and, if we control the outcomes, just like the CBT academics do, then won't we also get a slice of the financial and resource action? My personal reaction to this proposition remains one of ardent opposition, but its existence needs to be noted.

Won't there always be scandals in large-scale health systems? Haven't there always been? Isn't it just that now we find out about them?

This question is important in terms of the connections being made in some of the chapters between a neo-liberal and managerial perspective that drives a coach and horses through traditional expectations of health and social care. Nostalgia for a pre-Thatcher NHS, or suggesting that the NHS is simply not the right place to locate therapy services of any kind, strike me as almost equally problematic. If therapy is of value, then surely the NHS should be offering it? The problem, of course, is that a public sector therapy may ineluctably lead to docile and quashed clients. I am not sure what to think about it.

I worry about an alternative elitism that condemns all clients to independent services, whether offered by individuals or collectives and networks and with the descriptor 'community' added. Don't be deceived by this political rectitude, for these collectives and centres are often just a way of packaging relatively conventional one-to-one therapy.

Despite this caveat, it is certainly worth considering the benefits that national low-cost, and even free, therapy services might have to offer, also drawing on the existing 'therapy' that holds families, communities and civil society together already.

As is apparent, I feel personally divided about whether or not I want to see 'public sector' psychotherapy and counselling. I can see the strength of the arguments that says the state has no place in this kind of activity at all and should keep out. At the same time, in any realistic time scale, thinking about alternatives cannot possibly meet the needs that exist – or that we assume exist. In the long-term we are all dead.

Having asked and tested out partial responses to these questions, in order to constitute the Foreword for this book, I should like to add that, for me, reading it was a revelatory and reassuring experience. It was revelatory to realise that, despite our many differences of ideology, practice and personality, there is a coherent politics of psychotherapy and counselling abroad. This constitutes, crudely, the other side of the battle for the soul. This is what sets itself against the medical model, psychopharmacology and IAPT.

Earlier, I mentioned a campaign. Sometimes, and not only ironically, there has been talk recently (2014–2015) of a 'Campaign for Real Therapy'. Then some of us have started to refer to a 'Broad Front in Psychotherapy and Counselling' which would attend to all the big issues that this book so beautifully identifies. The book will be a part of whatever campaign does finally emerge. But the book is not only a contrarian work. What also comes over to me is the way in which love and compassion suffuse the various contributions. These authors know how to use their heads. Yet they also show that they have huge hearts (and bodies) as well. If you want to refer to the left-brain, be my guest.

A luta continua. 'We shall never surrender.'

Samuels' Letter to the Guardian, *27 October*
2007, www.theguardian.com

Psychotherapists have failed effectively to communicate their considerable concern over the Government's plan to train 3,500 Cognitive Behavioural Therapists. Partly this is because our leadership has thought something is better than nothing and that it would be irresponsible to let loose. Whatever the reason, we have allowed the proponents of CBT to caricature all other psychotherapies as delving unendingly into the patient's past and lacking any scientific validation as regards efficacy. Everyone knows the limitations of CBT – except, it would seem, the Government. The science is inadequate, the methods naive and manipulative, and the reluctance to engage with the key aspect of psychotherapy – the deep and complex relationship that develops between client and therapist – really very careless. Clients who enter CBT are approached in a mechanistic way, required to be passive and obedient. Hence what is going to be on offer is second class therapy for citizens deemed to be second class.

References

Norcross, J. (2011). *Psychotherapy relationships that work*. Oxford: Oxford University Press.
Veale, D. & Samuels, A. (2009). 'Improving access to psychological therapies – for and against. *Psychodynamic Practice*, 15(1), 41–56.

ACKNOWLEDGEMENTS

I wish to acknowledge the work of the contributors. Apart from the high standard of their scholarship, expertise and insight I would also like to acknowledge their professionalism and efficiency. I am an experienced Editor of professional and academic work in the field and their responsiveness and capacity to stick to deadlines has been second to none. In particular, I also wish to thank Dr Richard House for his enthusiasm, encouragement and help when I was putting together the proposal, Professor Andrew Samuels for writing the Foreword and Professor John Nuttall for reading the chapters and giving me a second opinion about the book. Finally, I wish to thank my partner, Fumiko Chikami, who has been a constant source of inspiration and encouragement and, as ever, is a welcome critic of my work.

1

INTRODUCTION

John Lees

The Tao which can be expressed in words is not the eternal Tao
the name which can be uttered is not its eternal name.
Without a name, it is the Beginning of Heaven and Earth.

Lao Tsu, Tao Te Ching[1]

I want to begin this opening chapter of the book by talking about fantasy and reality. We build a great part of our lives and aspirations out of the lives we would like to live rather than the lives that we are actually living (Phillips, 2013). The same thing could be said of mental health policy. The promises, predictions and rhetoric of policy makers, politicians and researchers are based on the reality that they want us to think we can live rather than the reality we actually live.

Over the years I have learnt that the most difficult thing in the world is to see reality as it is, as Lao Tsu noted some 2,500 years ago:

The Tao which can be expressed in words is not the eternal Tao
the name which can be uttered is not its eternal name.
Without a name, it is the Beginning of Heaven and Earth.

One of my primary aims as a counselling and psychotherapy (therapy) practitioner is to help clients to move ever closer to the mysterious and unfathomable ideal of seeing reality as it is. It is a driving force not only of my clinical work but also of my own development, my approach to the counselling and psychotherapy (therapy) profession and to life in general.

The future of the therapy profession is now in the balance. The commonly used term in the UK for therapy is now 'psychological therapy': the term used in the Government sponsored Improved Access to Psychological Therapies (IAPT) scheme in the NHS. The principles underpinning this scheme and its underlying managed care mind-set are beginning to determine the development of the profession as a whole and, in so doing, overwhelm the strong and varied traditions of therapy practice and research which have developed since the 1890s. Its rhetoric is based on fantasies about what can be achieved as opposed to realities, and it is essential that the transformative principles of counselling and psychotherapy are not forgotten as this 'revolution' takes place.

The managed care principles underpinning IAPT and 'psychological therapy' provide the starting point for this book. However its central aim is to argue for an approach to therapy based on the full range of discoveries that have been made since the origins of the profession for the benefit of the therapy profession itself, other professions, our clients and humanity at large. It will remind us that the profession did not begin with IAPT in 2006 but at the end of the nineteenth century. It is concerned with establishing a profession which is based on transformational, as well as managed care, principles.

The authors make frequent reference to neo-liberalism, managed care, evidence-based practice and the New Public Management (NPM) system. Neo-liberalism is based on *laissez faire* notions of leaving the market as free as possible to determine its own direction – and now the direction of public services including healthcare and therapy. It came to the fore in the Reagan administrations in United States and the Thatcher governments in United Kingdom in the 1980s. Business thinking began to rule in healthcare from the late 1980s and specifically in the therapy profession from 2006 in the form of the IAPT.

The NPM system in the UK began in 1983 when Margaret Thatcher's government commissioned Roy Griffiths to write a report on the management of the NHS. It espouses the three m's of managers, markets and measurement (Ferlie *et al.*, 1996) – four m's if you consider another central element: money. This was supplemented by the introduction of evidence-based medicine in 1992, which provided the research basis for this approach to healthcare.

NPM gives, at first, the impression that the practice is well-managed, orderly and transparent. However, this is far from the truth as demonstrated by a succession of scandals, subsequently leading to major public enquiries in the UK; for instance, the 2001 report on the Bristol Royal Infirmary (Kennedy, 2001) and the 2013 report on the Mid-Staffordshire NHS Foundation Trust (Francis, 2013). These reports have documented failures in the NPM systems. The problems have fallen into two categories: generalised systemic problems and problems arising from vagaries in human behaviour which affect the way in which professionals implement the systems. Indeed, there is a tension between these aspects of healthcare – between the varied interests of the institutions and the systems and the quality of care provided for patients and the unpredictability of the behaviour of people (Roberts, 2013). Moreover, the problems are persistent. In spite of the warnings and recommendations of the 2001 report, very little, if anything, had changed by the time of the 2013 report.

As regards the systems themselves, there are several problems. First, they are based on a task-based culture which prioritises targets over the quality of care (Fisher

& Freshwater, 2014): targets are 'pursued with a reckless disregard for the well-being and safety of patients' (Roberts, 2013). Second, Francis (2014) speaks about problems in reporting critical incidents; in particular, a 'lack of clarity into what constitutes an incident that should be reported'. He notes how reports of incidents led to little or no action. For instance, complaints by family members in Mid-Staffordshire did not produce changes (ibid., p. 74). Third, Tingle (2014), reviewing the effects of Francis' report, notes inconsistencies in measurement and evaluation. A survey of the response of the NHS Trusts to Francis, conducted by the Nuffield Trust stated that 'one of the case-study trusts, for example, had been flagged as "green" by the Care Quality Commission (CQC) for its performance on a specific quality measure, but had been failed by Monitor, which had declared the trust as being "in breach" for poor performance against the same dimension of quality'. Finally, Tingle (2014) also makes the general comment that the 'top down' systems of 'targets and finance rather than quality of care' seemed to be worse one year on, and the creation of a 'culture of compassion, support and mutual learning' was proving to be difficult to implement as long as management was seen as external and punitive.

As regards human behaviour, Francis (2014) speaks about defensiveness among carers and managers. For instance, managers defend themselves against failures to meet targets, which is not surprising since many of them fear that they will lose their jobs if they do not achieve targets (Roberts, 2013). Francis (2014) also reports cases of staff victimisation while Newdick and Danbury (2014) speak about a 'failure to recognise' patients' 'humanity and individuality and to respond to them with sensitivity, compassion and professionalism'.

A limitation of the Francis report is that it does not engage with the strengths and expertise of health practitioners. The report only addressed problems with the systems themselves. Recommendations about practitioner behaviour included such admirable statements as the need for practitioners to 'contribute to a safer, committed and compassionate and caring service' and for care to be provided by a 'caring, compassionate and committed staff, working within a common culture' (Francis, 2013). But it did not have a plan to do this. There was no theoretical framework and no methodology of practitioner research. Transformational therapy-inspired practice and research methodologies can help with the problems. This book can contribute to this as it draws on a wealth of practitioner expertise in the field of therapy practice and research.

An underlying concern of the book is that we are perpetuating the same systems in the therapy profession in the form of IAPT in spite of such well-documented failures. Clearly, the supporters of IAPT consider that their approach to managed care and evidence-based practice is the best approach to psychological therapy research and practice. They see the scheme as building up an 'integrated and high quality psychological therapy provision' and argue that it will 'strive to make these services safe, effective and successful in improving mental wellbeing, reducing stigma and health inequalities' thereby 'making the United Kingdom a world leader in psychological therapies' (New Savoy Conferences, 2012). This policy is laudable.

The scheme is to provide psychological therapy on a scale that has never been done before. But it can be enhanced by research done by therapists in several ways. First, it can contribute to the quality (as opposed to the quantity) of the care provided by IAPT. Second, it can help to integrate the findings of 100 years of psychotherapy research into the scheme. Third, it can go beyond the rhetoric and open up space for independent thought and reflection about the full range of therapeutic possibilities. Fourth, it can prevent a gradual spreading of the principles under-pinning the scheme, as a result of its extension into such services as student counselling and other aspects of counselling and psychotherapy provision.

Many of the chapters in this book refer to the fantasy nature of the scheme. I have chosen a short sample of these phrases:

- whilst National Institute for Health and Care Excellence (NICE) recognises many of the issues concerning its methodology, it ends up acting as if they don't exist;
- approaches to therapy today 'take clients' minds off their problems rather than attempting to help them work through 'what is bothering them';
- there are enduring efforts to impose symbolic order on an anxiety that can never be completely managed;
- IAPT operates in a virtuality, focusing on performativity and surveillance rather than real encounters;
- there is an 'unrecognised, imaginary or fantastic basis of much public health policy-making';
- the 'evidence based' research culture is 'a series of dogmas which fuel a fantasy of discovering a "perfect" all-encompassing understanding of how we function together';
- there is a fantasy that 'everything that happens in our world must be safe';
- it 'seems particularly absurd to think of many therapists all trying to "provide" the same "intervention" in a standardized fashion'.

Another theme running through the book is that the managed care dominant discourse, the dominant metanarrative, the juggernaut that is driving the thera-peutic, caring and educational professions (and basically the world) forward is not only built on fantasies but also on exercising power over people. With this in mind I collated another set of phrases which are interspersed throughout the book:

- the state is using psychotherapy, psychoanalysis and counselling as a form of social control;
- it creates a climate of 'distraction and fear';
- it is 'the culture of monitor, watch, control which chillingly echoes the grim predictions of Orwell';
- there is a tendency for impersonal systems to determine 'what is or is not permitted to occur within the organisation, between staff and within psychological treatment';

- the systems are heightening 'anxiety levels by over-controlling the policy and procedural structure';
- one day there may be 'a CCTV camera in the corner of the therapy room ceiling, ready to alert the Therapy Police to break down the door';
- there is 'a critical shift in the locus of power away from the professional autonomy of practitioners themselves';
- the NHS and IAPT are perhaps the last vestiges of Weberian bureaucracy in the current neo-liberal age.

The chapters are divided into three broad overlapping parts: the context of therapy (Mainly Context), the influence of NPM and IAPT (Mainly IAPT) and clinical practice (Mainly Practice). Each part highlights the principal focus but also includes elements of the other areas as well.

In Part I Del Loewenthal, Stuart Morgan-Ayrs and William Bento look at the broader context of therapy and research today. Del Loewenthal speaks about the restriction of our freedoms in therapy, as in life in general, and how this limits the 'subversive' nature of therapy which takes place in a 'confidential space where clients can explore anything that comes to their minds'. He challenges us to think about the futility of theory and suggests that we re-vision therapy as a cultural practice. He also outlines the flaws in the systems and approaches of research which are increasingly bearing down on therapists and oppressing them, whether they are aware of it or not (such as randomised controlled trials, NICE and IAPT) and refers to the commodification of therapy. This echoes some of the themes in the chapter by Stuart Morgan-Ayrs. The main focus of this chapter is the drive towards regulation in all its forms, the dangers of therapy becoming 'highly formulaic and inauthentic' and, even worse, the 'sterilization' of therapy and the 'creation of a specific box which is pre-defined for the therapist to live in'. He looks at how this mind-set, which is beginning to dominate the therapy profession, severely limits therapeutic possibilities by becoming too defined and colonising the minds of practitioners (Foucauldian subjectification).

William Bento points out that, as in many aspects of our lives today, new developments, such as managed care, began in the United States before they came to the United Kingdom. Managed care in the United States can be traced back to 1973, ten years before the systems were introduced into the United Kingdom in 1983. The language is different – and there is of course no National Health Service – but the principles are the same. A central idea is the Health Maintenance Organizations (HMOs) which exercise a great deal of power over practitioners. The chapter includes such familiar themes as the dominance of money, with an emphasis on dollars saved as opposed to quality of care, the 'disparity between the medical science oriented approach and the humanistic/holistic views found in psychological and sociological paradigms' and the problem of treating symptoms rather than seeing the client as a 'developing human being'.

Part II of the book consists of chapters by Ian Simpson, Rosemary Rizq, Jay Watts and John Nuttall, all of whom look at the limitations of the managed care systems in the United Kingdom and the IAPT scheme in particular based on their direct experience of these systems. Ian Simpson, drawing on his experience of managing a therapy service, looks at the process of dismantling a service and the effect of this on practitioners and their clients. He describes how the service had been managed using the therapeutic principles of containment and holding and how the service was 'actively undermined' by the business and target orientation of the neo-liberal NPM system. Like many chapters in the book, he highlights how the realities of the political, cultural and social context on the service were denied and led to what he calls the denigration of the human. He examines splits which develop between the objectives of managers and administrators and the practitioners running and working in the service.

Rosemary Rizq looks at how the policies of managed care with its 'growing demand for transparency, accountability and governance' is driven by anxiety 'at both individual and organisational levels because they bring us into unwilling contact with our own abjected vulnerability'. Using a case example, she shows how the realities of human suffering are 'deemed to be repulsive or untouchable' and how contemporary managed care systems constitute a 'symbolic attempt to gain mastery over feelings unconsciously deemed to be abject reminders of the body'. Jay Watts draws on her experience of working in an early IAPT site and supervising many IAPT practitioners. She demonstrates the gap between the ideals of IAPT and the reality and shows how 'its promises', far from achieving what they purport to achieve 'may actually increase the level of anguish in society'. She examines the privileging of CBT, the lack of thorough assessments, high-dropout rates and the central role of the lightly trained PWPs (psychological wellbeing practitioners) and suggests that IAPT is predominantly concerned with making the 'state run smoothly' and moulding the self 'so as to become attractive to the market'. John Nuttall, Chair of the Trustees of a major IAPT service provider, examines the clash of values between the service and the IAPT scheme. He shows how the challenges of IAPT were successfully negotiated by the service and presents a way into the future based on a uniquely psychotherapeutic approach to values.

In Part III of the book, John Lees, Nick Totton and Richard House look mainly at practice and build up a perspective on therapy which presents a different approach from managed care. In my chapter, I look at some key aspects of man-aged care and contrast them to relational psychotherapy and creative methodologies, both of which developed in the same period as managed care and evidence-based practice. I demonstrate the transformational power of these marginalised discourses and show how they have the potential to bring about social change. Nick Totton builds his chapter around several themes, including the notion of therapy as an inherently risky undertaking and therapy as a practice of truth. He looks at risk from the point of view of ethics and addresses the way in which ethical principles are turned into laws that need to be policed leading to defensive practice. In contrast he sees the true essence of ethics as developing a healthy sense of rightness arising out of a unique intersubjective co-construction between the therapist and client. He also addresses the uniqueness of each therapy contract, surveillance in therapy and discusses a way forward for the profession. Richard House draws a distinction between therapy as manualisation and therapy as a 'spontaneous co-creation'. The current direction of the therapy profession (and modern culture in general) socialises us into 'thinking like a state'. It creates a therapy which is based on 'managerialist imperatives and administrative bureaucratic interests', is audit driven, concentrates on getting people back to work, is defensive and can only support the status quo. Yet he also speaks of a different approach to therapy that embraces 'ambiguity, not knowing, the intuitive and the mysterious', is relationally orientated, is holistic and relies on the client's capacity to self-heal.

In the final chapter I bring together some of the threads of the book. I look at the challenges we are facing today and the nature of the future we are creating. I show that the book is not just about critiquing managed care and IAPT but about looking at innovatory approaches to clinical practice and research, which stand outside the 'evidence based' approaches of IAPT. I thus open up the possibility of working towards a more balanced and grounded way forward for the counselling and psychotherapy profession and for the way we think about psychological problems. I also show how the book demonstrates that transformational practice and research is an ongoing project with many discoveries still to make.

At the beginning of this introduction I looked at the issues of fantasy and power in healthcare and their influence on psychological therapy today. The book elaborates on these themes and provides much more as well. It presents a constructive way forward in spite of the challenges facing the therapy profession today. It demonstrates how therapists have the capacity to break through the rhetoric and obfuscations of IAPT managed care and, in so doing, understand what is *really* happening in IAPT. More importantly, it shows that therapy is still fresh and alive and has the capacity for innovation and individual and social transformation. The profession did not just develop its clinical base in the twentieth century, with its proliferation of theories once and for all and then come to a halt. It is still developing new ideas and has many new discoveries to make. Its creative power has not diminished. It is important to recognise this in order to create a balanced profession in which managed care and the views expressed in this book could engage in constructive dialogue with each other. Moreover its ongoing discoveries are relevant to other healthcare and human science professions and not just counselling and psychotherapy.

Note

1   Translated by Lionel Giles in 1904.

References

Ferlie, E., Ashburner, L., Fitzgerald, L. & Pettigrew, A. (1996). *New public management in action*. Oxford: Oxford University Press.

Fisher, P. & Freshwater, D. (2014). Towards compassionate care through aesthetic rationality. *Scandinavian Journal of Caring Sciences*, 28(4): 767–74.

Francis, R. (2013). Report of the Mid Staffordshire NHS Foundation Trust Public Inquiry Retrieved 9 December 2013 from: www.midstaffspublicinquiry.com/report.

Francis, R. (2014). Culture, compassion and clinical neglect – probity in the NHS after Mid Staffordshire. *Journal of Medical Ethics*. Retrieved February 2015 from: http://jme.bmj. com/content/early/2014/01/07/medethics-2013-101462.extract.

Kennedy, I. (2001). The report of the public inquiry into children's heart surgery at the Bristol Royal Infirmary 1984–1995: Learning from Bristol. Retrieved February 2015 from: http://webarchive.nationalarchives.gov.uk/+/www.dh.gov.uk/en/Publicationsand statistics/Publications/PublicationsPolicyAndGuidance/DH_4005620.

Newdick, C. & Danbury, C. (2014). Culture, compassion and clinical neglect: Probity in the NHS after Mid Staffordshire. *Journal of Medical Ethics*. doi: 10.1136/medethics-2012-101048.

New Savoy Conferences. (2012). The New Savoy declaration 2012. Retrieved June 2014 from: www.newsavoypartnership.org/docs/NSP-Revised-Declaration-for-web.pdf.

Phillips, A. (2013). *Missing out*. London: Penguin Books.

Roberts, D. J. (2013). The Francis report on the Mid-Staffordshire NHS Foundation Trust: Putting patients first. *Transfusion Medicine*, 23, 73–6.

Tingle, J. (2014). The Francis report: One year on. *British Journal of Nursing*, 23(5), 284–5.

PART I

Mainly context

2

THERAPY AS CULTURAL, POLITICALLY INFLUENCED PRACTICE

Del Loewenthal

Introduction

Is it true that now psychotherapists are being asked to comply with an evidence-based practice that has been constructed to favour approaches that do not enable clients and patients to explore meaning in depth? In this chapter it will be argued that a revolution has already started whereby the freedom as to what is carried out by psychotherapists and explored by their clients/patients has, as with so many areas of our lives, become severely restricted. It would appear that professional bodies of psychotherapists are increasingly attempting to go along with this audit culture that is considered here to be, at best, pseudo-science. It will be argued that the result is that psychological therapies have lost their way into unwittingly becoming agents of the state. This process, it will be argued, has greatly reduced not only the choice that is being offered to patients and clients but the extent to which psychological therapies can be essentially subversive and can provide a confidential space where clients have the freedom to explore anything that comes to their minds. An illustration of how such changes come about is explored through how the National Institute for Health and Care Excellence (NICE) attempts to measure the effects of psychotherapy. However, in contrast to the audit culture of New Public Management, the nature of our work, which we seem in danger of forgetting, will first be considered before examining how its erroneous measurement is catastrophically changing what was originally thought of as our project. It will be argued that we are in a war and there may just be a chance that psychotherapy can wake up and do something before it is too late. Overall the concern is that, regarding mental health, psychiatry and psychology are based on false theoretical foundations, and our governments seem determined that psychotherapy should follow suit.

Didn't Freud, Klein and others first discover practices? Subsequently, they and others devised theories (now over 600 of them) to explain these practices. More recently, certain types of research to justify these theories have been the order of the day. It is suggested here that psychotherapy, psychoanalysis and counselling have no theoretical foundations, and their associated theories, although they can be helpful, are not foundational and that, perhaps, to consider them as such is a delusion. In which case isn't it possible for a theory to have implications and that to consider any theory, individually or collectively, as the foundation or as an application, as might particularly be seen in cases of manualisation, is based on a false premise? Hence the following questions: Is psychotherapy first and foremost a practice? Are theories more attempts to explain practice or is theory the basis of psychotherapeutic practice? Do changes in this practice have more to do with changes in our culture that in turn lead us to be more interested in different theories? What are the forces in our society that make cognitive behavioural therapy (CBT) so prevalent to the extent that such scientifically very questionable notions of using Randomised Controlled Trials (RCTs) as a so-called evidence base are used for the state-sanctioning of therapeutic practice?

This article is in four sections: The first looks at psychotherapies (and research) as cultural practices, the second studies the workings of the NICE in relation to psychotherapy, the third looks at what changes in our society may have given rise to the current prevalence of CBT, and the fourth considers what, if anything, can be done?

So, is the questioning of CBT just a part of a process of denial from some psychotherapists who aren't in the ascendancy and are taking it out on the state? Are all these different psychotherapeutic notions really to keep the psychotherapist occupied while something else therapeutically useful can happen? Can any modality really claim to be the only game in town?

There is the particularly important question as to whether psychotherapists can actually diagnose and treat as in the medical model. The medical model (or RCTs) with regard to physical medicine are not being questioned here. To give a personal example, when I broke my wrist I had no quarrel with the doctor's implicit understanding of what I wanted my healed wrist to be like. But if I break my heart can anyone, let alone a technician, tell me what my desire should be? However, it is important to acknowledge NICE's excellent work in attempting to get drug companies to report all their RCTs rather than just the successful ones (which perhaps shows what it is possible, at times, to get away with when using the term 'RCT'). Yet isn't using RCTs for mental health an absurdity? Isn't there also a strong case for more public scrutiny of the evidence base of the Diagnostic and Statistical Manual (DSM)? Not only is there a case for suggesting that theorising is scandalous, as my colleague James Davies (2013) among others has suggested but also equally scandalous is a situation where any psychotropic medication is only required to be tested once after eight weeks, when people are on it for more than eight weeks and, in too many cases, for the rest of their lives? It is being suggested here that we do have Richard Layard (2005) to thank for getting successive governments to accept the use of talking therapies over drug therapies. But what of our own classification of different modalities? Can any really be scientifically proven to be better than another? Will there be sufficient choice so that those who want to explore personal (rather than medical) meaning, the importance of which has been described, for example, by those recovering from a psychiatric diagnosis, can do so? (Cotton & Loewenthal, 2015).

Psychotherapy as a cultural practice

The place of practice at the heart of psychotherapy and counselling (Loewenthal, 2011) is being argued for here. This aim can be seen as stretching from the time of Pyrrhonian scepticism to, more recently, the writings of Wittgenstein, where what we do can be understood to be more about the activities in which we participate with our clients. There is therefore an increasing body of opinion showing the futility of theory as the basis of the psychological therapies (Heaton, 2013; Frie & Orange, 2009; Brown & Stenner, 2009) and, with it, what is currently regarded as research. But psychological therapies are also cultural practices, and we are attempting to reformulate an understanding of meaning as contextual and emerging through a meeting of the psychological therapist and client.

Thus, how we understand such emerging meaning will be mediated by cultural practices through the mixture of ideas that permeate our society in any period. An attempt is therefore being made here to describe a potential cultural movement that currently pervades and, I think in some ways pragmatically and strategically, that CBT so helpfully meets for some. However, with regard to false foundations it is not only CBT but any therapies, whether they be humanistic, existential or psychoanalytic, which become totalising moves and are potentially violent as they encompass the individual completely within theoretical frame-ups. At best, such theories are secondary and, while they may have implications, they can never provide a foundation to the primacy of practice.

In any meeting we are involved with such aspects as talk, ritual and gesture. Yet one does not do it based on theory; it is a practice, a cultural practice that can change within a culture and can be different between cultures. If one theorises about practice, it is done outside of practice; it is different. Also, one might end up theorising about the bone and muscle properties of the hand and arm or even the mouth as one gestures or speaks, but it won't help much.

Isn't it the same with all psychotherapies – are they not practices which Freud and others later tried to theorise about? But doesn't this theory come from somewhere other than the practice that precedes it? And isn't it a different kind of knowledge? Also, isn't most of what is so frequently taught as psychology unhelpful here – learning, for example, about the ear or the larynx doesn't usually help us as psychotherapists, does it? Are counselling and psychotherapeutic theories any better? Does Bion (1962) come closest to theorising practice with his system 'O' (the ineffable: the unknowable or ultimate truth)? Or is Polanyi (1966) better with his notion of tacit knowledge, which by definition can never be explicitly defined? There again, to what extent is well-being or the good to do with the knowledge derived from research?

How we are with patients/clients might be seen as an act of judgment, and we might reflect on what we have said, but does that make us practitioner researchers? Not if we take research to mean achieving generalisation through some systematic approach.

Don't psychotherapists already have their own way of being thoughtful about their work in, for example, taking it to clinical supervision and writing and presenting papers? RCTs are so inappropriate and against the very nature of what for many is the therapeutic enterprise (see for example House & Loewenthal, 2008).

Research as a cultural practice

So psychotherapy as a cultural practice has, or attempts, to obtain, legitimacy through whatever it provides for that culture. Often these days, empirical research is the legitimising tool, and this more recently has to be 'evidence based' without having to consider what the evidence of, for example, love or intimacy is. Is research another cultural practice? As one person who took part in a significant RCT said when I asked what her research had to do with truth and justice, 'Not much' she said, 'but I got my modality accepted'. We then, of course, get researcher allegiance to boot (Budge, Baardseth, Wampold & Flückiger, 2010; Munder, Brütsch, Leonhart, Gerger & Barth, 2013).

Research is what all psychotherapeutic professional bodies are now pushing their members and trainees to do. Yet isn't this another cultural practice that is linked to legitimising changes in our culture (McNamee, 2010)? I have never understood how anyone with a basic school qualification in mathematics could ever claim that RCTs could be the gold standard for so much psychotherapy research. Indeed, because of the work that I was commissioned to do by the United Kingdom Council for Psychotherapy (UKCP), which also appeared as 'Scrutinising NICE' (see Guy, Loewenthal, Thomas & Stephenson, 2012), questions were asked in the House and fundamental flaws were acknowledged by the previous and current head of NICE. It then appeared there was an attempt to find another method whereby psychotherapeutic modalities could be objectively evaluated while RCTs looked set to continue only temporarily as the order of the day. (I shall say more about NICE and the current situation in a moment.) But first what research is really of use to us as practitioners? From what I can see, very little if we think in terms of generalisation. Indeed, for those of us interested in research, it seems the most important aspect of our work is to remind people how the consequences of applying any of it to our practices may be more detrimental than beneficial. Isn't Physis or Phusis what comes out of its self (McNamee, 2014; Shotter, 2005, 2014)? But now the measuring instruments determine the therapy and as Vygotsky (1986) states, we are shaped by the tools and instruments we come to use.

There is a changing fashion in what we regard as research – what was acceptable as a doctorate some years ago can be different from what is acceptable in the same discipline today, where empirical, positivistic research is in the ascendancy. Theoretical explorations are rarely now considered by our professional bodies as research or, indeed, by an increasing number of university departments where one will be lucky if it is classified instead by what is regarded as the less significant term 'scholarship'. Now quantitative empirical studies rule the day.

So what has research got to do with thoughtful practice? I have been interested in different types of research and was indeed the Chair of UKCP's first Research Committee, but I regard most of what is now research in the psychological therapies, whether it be quantitative or qualitative, as more often than not being far worse than a waste of time. Indeed as Merleau-Ponty (2002[1962]) has said, sometimes if one attempts to take away the mystery, one can take away the thing itself. Furthermore, for those, who like myself, once thought qualitative research might be more helpful

> . . . rethinking humanist ontology is key in what comes after humanist qualitative methodology. If we cease to privilege knowing over being; if we refuse positivist and phenomenological assumptions about the nature of lived experience and the world; if we give up representational and binary logics; if we see language, the human, and the material not as separate entities mixed together but as completely imbricated 'on the surface' – if we do all that and 'more', it will open up – will qualitative inquiry as we know it be possible?'
>
> *(Lather & St. Pierre, 2013, p. 630)*

Or to put it another way, as it happened when that French Minster of Health was under pressure to evaluate psychoanalysis and replied: 'Psychoanalysis is something else and we should let it be' (Snell, 2007).

I have previously used the name 'post-existentialism' in an attempt to describe a potential cultural moment whereby psychological therapies can be considered to at least start with practice and counter the hegemony of training technicians as psychological therapists perhaps to oil the wheels of our increasingly dominant managerialist culture (see, for example, Loewenthal, 2010).

So doesn't research, in attempting to either legitimise theories and/or provide a means of accountability within state funded practices, take us away from what was the essence of psychotherapeutic practice? For example, whatever the name, is it possible for us to have an approach to psychological therapies that attempts to let us experience our alienation, which many would see as inevitable in a capitalist society (for example, Blauner, 1964), in the hope that we may still be able, individually and collectively, to do more about it? (When I was a student we all read and talked about alienation. Now we seem to be so alienated that this is no longer possible.) With the psychological therapies, aren't we meant to open up a space where people, if they want to, can confidentially explore any thought, dream, fantasy, or problem with others, including those in authority? Indeed shouldn't psychological therapies be essentially subversive? Is it really possible for the state to endorse us to allow clients/patients to explore meanings in their specific contexts, without ignoring the work of the post-modernists, the psychoanalysts or the political? Or was that just about okay previously for a few but now, when there are over one million people per year in this country having therapy (Chunn, 2013), are previous freedoms too great a risk for the powers that be in terms of social control? Is that why there is this extraordinary recent interest in the provision and controlling of psychological therapies?

NICE work if you can get it: Can you get how NICE works?

There is also the question that perhaps 'it's not such nice work even if you can get 'it'! (see for example Rizq, 2013). However, it was hoped that some people might read this as 'Can you get how NICE works?'

In 'Scrutinising NICE' (Guy *et al.*, 2012) we provided the following overview: 'Consequences for patient choice of NICE guidelines implemented via Improving Access to Psychological Therapies (IAPT)':

- NICE's methodology has been inappropriately applied to the talking therapies.
- The relevance of the assumptions that underpin NICE's preferred research method, RCTs, is questioned.
- While NICE recognises many of the issues raised concerning its methodology, it is *acting* as though they don't exist.
- The current process works in favour of some therapies (e.g. CBT) and puts others at an unreasonable disadvantage.
- NICE should adopt a pluralist approach to research methodologies, following the lead of the American Psychological Association (APA).

It would appear that successive heads of NICE have recognised the inappropriateness of RCTs but don't know what to replace it with. For those not familiar with the process of NICE, we think it is important that you note their language. It is embedded in a model of biological medicine where patients' experiences (*symptoms*) are indicative of underlying *conditions*, which need to be *diagnosed* in order for an appropriate *treatment* to be *prescribed* (a language which I imagine a few psychological therapists warm to and others don't). What happens is:

- A '*condition*' on which to issue guidelines about *treatment options is selected*.
- A 'Guideline Development Group (GDG)' is created.
- Research conducted on 'interventions' for participants who have been '*diagnosed*' with the '*condition*' is examined giving primacy to those studies which have used RCTs.

NICE seems to recognise concerns about such constructions of depression as a clinical condition, but all their guidelines are based on evidence gathered around patients who have been diagnosed with a relevant condition. As Bentall (2009) points out, such diagnostic systems have no evidence of usefulness.

Regarding NICE's GDGs, 'the exact composition of the GDG should be tailored to the topic covered by the clinical guideline. It should reflect the range of stakeholders and groups whose professional activities or care will be covered by the guidelines' (NICE, 2009: p. 29). One of the problems here is that if stakeholders do not recognise the use of diagnoses, then their 'research evidence' is not included. Some psychoanalytic schools use diagnoses in a more metaphorical use of the medical model, here for example 'the person's individuality eventually becomes more impressive than his or her conformity with an abstraction (Hoffman, 2009). However, a significant number of psychotherapists, researchers and doctors do not believe diagnoses of mental health conditions are valid. For example, with regard to psychiatry:

> Fully realised, these criticisms of the evidence supporting professionalised mental health services and practices have profound implications. At face value they can be read *'There is no conclusive science supporting claims that any of the psycho-pharmaceuticals work as claimed, and when they do help, it is as likely as not that "help" is the result of complex phenomena not indistinguishable from placebo'* and *'Useful outcomes of a psychological therapy are primarily the result of a helpful relationship, rather than the result of any identifiable psychotherapeutic technique'*. If these conclusions were to be widely acknowledged … much of what conventional mental health services are commissioned to do would have to be seen as acts of faith rather than fact. In the event few have reacted to *Beyond the Current Paradigm* with any rebuttal of these underpinning conclusions, despite the fact that it was published in the house magazine of the Royal College of Psychiatrists.
>
> *(Middleton, 2015)*

But back to NICE. NICE seem to be, on the one hand, aware of some of the problems; so for example, it is stated in their GDG for Depression that they *'considered it important to acknowledge the uncertainty inherent in our current understanding of depression and its classification, and that assuming a false categorical certainty is likely to be unhelpful and, even worse, damaging'* (NICE, 2009, pp. 23–4). However, despite these factors, NICE only seriously considered research evidence conducted using participants with depression as a firm 'diagnosis' (e.g. NICE, 2009, p. 262).

So who in fact are the stakeholders who play an essential part in NICE's recommendations, which includes 'where evidence is lacking the guidelines incorporate statements and recommendations based upon consolidated statements developed by the GDG' (NICE, 2009, p. 12). The GDG for Depression comprises: Chair: Consultant Psychiatrist, Psychiatrists: 2, Psychological Therapist: 1, Psychotherapist: 1, Clinical Psychologists: 2, GPs: 2, Nurses: 2, Pharmacist: 1, Service Users: 2, Carer: 1 (15 in total incl. Chair).

In fact, at the time of publishing our work on 'Scrutinising NICE' (Guy *et al.*, 2012), and unfortunately little seems to have changed since, an overall review of the composition of the GDGs that produced the clinical guidelines on anxiety, depression in adults and schizophrenia showed that 6.7 per cent were psychological therapists and 33 per cent from the medical profession. Furthermore, 36 per cent were from the National Collaborating Centre for Mental Health. And who are they? They are drawn from: 'a partnership between the Royal College of Psychiatry and the British Psychological Society's Centre for Outcome Research and Effectiveness' (NICE, 2009, p. 13), whose director is a clinical psychologist. You might say 'at least we have a psychotherapist and a psychological therapist on the GDG for Depression to attempt to counterbalance this'. However, one is a Consultant Cognitive Behavioural Psychotherapist and is the Chair of the New Savoy Partnership and the other 'holds psychodynamic psychotherapy and supervision qualifications'. It would appear that the only psychotherapeutic advice this GDG receives is from the Chair of the New Savoy Partnership, a Consultant Cognitive Behavioural Psychotherapist, and those clinical psychologists from the National Collaborating Centre for Mental Health who are 'committed to CBT type research, closely involved in developing NICE guidelines' (Mollon, 2009). Yet psychological therapists appear to have been regarded as one homogeneous professional group. It *matters* that NICE appears not to have ensured adequate representation of psychotherapists.

> Where evidence is lacking, the guidelines incorporate statements and recommendations based upon the consensus statements developed by the GDG.
>
> *(NICE, 2009, p. 12)*

Again, as we report in Guy *et al.* (2012), NICE appears to state some of the limitations but doesn't act on it. For example, 'the importance of organising care in order to support and encourage a good therapeutic relationship is at times as important as the specific treatments offered' (NICE, 2009, pp. 12–13).

'It is difficult to determine whether or not the benefits. . .resulted specifically from the therapy or the prolonged contact with the therapist during that time' (NICE, 2009, p. 162).

Indeed as stated by Pilgrim *et al.* (2009, p. 244) *'the quality of the relationship consistently predicts outcome, independent of the espoused model or condition being treated'*. So how come the so-called gold standard research method, RCTs, is precisely one that attempts to neutralise the effect of a particular therapist?

What has really led to the current prevalence of CBT?

What happened to those in government such as that French Minister of Health who stated 'psychic suffering is neither measurable nor open to evaluation' (Snell, 2007)? In this review of Jacques-Alain Miller (2006) 'L'Anti-Livre noir de la psychanalyse', Snell also writes:

> For where the British psychoanalytic establishment has, for the most part, been anxious to go along with the challenge to produce 'evidence' and demonstrate 'treatment efficacy', the francophone world – as represented here, at least – will have none of it. In . . . the book, Yves Cartuyvels, an eminent Belgian professor of law who has spent his professional life examining the nature of evidence, refutes the claims of cognitive-behavioural therapy to

be founded – 'objectively' and 'scientifically' – in solid evidence. Such claims are mere scientism; they rest on 'a superannuated conception of science as the measure of ultimate truth' and a naïve nineteenth-century scientific positivism: 'the epistemology of science might as well not have bothered underlining, as it has been doing for many years, the social construction of science, or describing the interplay of its actors, and the interests and values behind the practice of science'. These claims also necessitate a refusal to accept that a patient might choose 'a rationality other than scientific rationality in response to psychic malaise'. In any case what, Cartuyvels asks, is 'effective' in the field of mental health? 'The suppression of a symptom? Help with living with a symptom? Who fixes and defines the thresholds of effectiveness? Science? The therapist? The subject? Are these thresholds the same from one individual to another, from one kind of suffering to another?'

(Snell, 2007 pp. 231–9)

Somehow notions of evidence and accountability within state-funded practices have come to ascendancy in a way that may serve certain vested interest groups, rather than necessarily all clients.

In concluding our previous research on 'Scrutinising NICE' (2012), we summarised that while NICE recognises many of the issues concerning its methodology, it ends up acting as if they don't exist. UKCP's lobbying based on our work resulted in the new Chair of NICE making them a commitment to review the way NICE assesses the evidence base for the psychological therapies.

It would appear that subsequently NICE decided that a review was not required. This is despite UKCP working with others, including the British Psychoanalytic Council (BPC), the Psychotherapists from the Royal College of Psychiatrists, British Association for Counselling and Psychotherapy (BACP) and Association of Child Psychotherapists (ACP), and submitting a joint consultation response on NICE's guideline manual. For many the consequences are that patient choice is greatly reduced, and there is likely to be decreasing work opportunities for psychological therapists who are not accredited to use sanctioned, evidence-based modalities. So how has this come about, and what if anything can be done?

Importantly, some would suggest (e.g. Harvey, 2007; Verhaeghe, 2014) we are in the age of neo-liberalism. The implications of this and how we might respond to this are now considered drawing on my book *Critical Psychotherapy, Psychoanalysis and Counselling: Implications for Practice* (Loewenthal, 2015). The prevailing climate appears to facilitate the growth of manualised, state-regulated therapies, aimed at taking clients' minds off their concerns using 'technicians' (Parker & Revelli, 2008; Mace, Rowland, Evans, Schroder & Halstead, 2009). As one IAPT evaluator has put it, there has been a transformation in practice in recent years, moving from a 'cottage industry to a factory-based production line' (Parry, Blackmore, Beecroft & Booth, 2010) with equally disruptive effects for practitioners. Perhaps psychotherapists should consider their modality, whatever it is, and wonder about the use of, often so-called 'science' in the pursuit of vested interests' notions of progress and authority.

We are also in an era where, through Edward Snowden's revelations (Harding, 2014) that our telephone calls and emails are monitored in the name of internal security, there would appear to have been a significant shift from accepting talking therapies as essentially both confidential and subversive and inevitably being located on the edges of our society. Instead, with practices and trainings becoming *increasingly* registered, regulated and incorporated into mainstream society, the result is the constant risk assessment of this confidentiality (Loewenthal, 2014). A growing pervasive audit culture and limited notions of evidence-based practice, involving some dubious claims to be 'scientific', can be seen as legitimising this change. Yet isn't this more to do with the attempts of those in power at a particular time to determine what is and is not science? As Foucault states, 'if we ask what is, in its very general form, the kind of division governing our will to knowledge – then we may well discern something like a system of exclusion (historical, modifiable, institutionally constraining)' (Foucault, 1971 pp. 7–30).

Our students are increasingly seeing their training as a commodity they are purchasing as customers rather than as a personal exploration. A concern here was, and still is, if the notion of critical psychotherapy, psychoanalysis and counselling is established it will become a minority module on mainstream programmes. The implication therefore is that it will become by definition primarily 'uncritical', but the 'critical' add-on will allow for a notion of democracy and, perhaps, for what is becoming an illusion of academic freedom. What is new, however, is the increasing extent of the state's involvement in purchasing/providing specific psychological therapies, alongside our new era of neo-liberalism and the New Public Management with its audit culture and its 'Markets, Managers and Measurement' (Barzelay, 2001; Gruening, 2001).

There seem to be two parallel developments taking place in the talking therapies. First, we have neo-liberalism that encourages 'the privatisation of everything public and the commercialisation of all things private' (Barber, 2000). This affects our relationships (Verhaeghe, 2014), including what is meant by the notion of public service and how we attempt to educate. It can be argued that the introduction of 'New Public Management' provides a smokescreen for such privatisation. However, in the name of safeguarding the public, the state is simultaneously tightening its grip on the psychological therapies. Certainly there have been some abuses by psychotherapists as well as doctors, nurses and other professionals, but isn't there now far more managerial abuse with far fewer checks and balances than previously?

Verhaeghe (2014) has argued that neo-liberalism has brought out the worst in us, in which case where do psychotherapy, psychoanalysis and counselling place themselves, if they can, in relation to these cultural changes? Can 'critical' psychotherapy, psychoanalysis and counselling provide an alternative space within this neo-liberal culture where the talking therapies are increasingly becoming agents of social control? Or will the talking therapies only be allowed to survive if we don't rock the neo-liberalist boat too much? The market that was supposed to emancipate us appears instead to have offered atomisation and loneliness

(Verhaeghe, 2014). So what of 'the common good 'in both this and our work as talking therapists? Furthermore, while we, as talking therapists, see people whose work is alienating and mainly offers extrinsic rewards, isn't even our own work becoming one where '[t]he workplace has been overwhelmed by a mad, Kafkaesque infrastructure of assessments, monitoring, measuring, surveillance and audits, centrally directed and rigidly planned' (Monbiot, 2014)?

The Layard report (2005) and the recommendations for the talking therapies from the National Institute for Health and Care Excellence (NICE, 2009) have possibly had the greatest effect on psychotherapy, psychoanalysis and counselling in the UK. First, the Layard report has been influential in that it has convinced successive governments in placing the case for the talking therapies in contrast to pharmaceutical interventions. Second, governments are increasingly taking mental health needs seriously. The IAPT national programme provides for mental health on a population-based basis, and so the government's role becomes central to the training, provision and delivery of talking therapy. This results in a focus on what many see as narrowly defined evidence-based practices. Can we really provide evidence of psychotherapists' abilities to enhance their clients' capacities for such aspects as intimacy and love, without at best something similar to the measurement of a good poem, as in the film *The Dead Poet's Society*? Favoured approaches tend to meet the imposed measurement systems; these seem to be those approaches that take clients' minds off their problems rather than attempting to help them work through what is bothering them. These favoured approaches are those talking therapies where the evidence base has been established through RCTS, and the public are encouraged to seek these out. We can hopefully only imagine the incredulity of future generations, given the questions over how appropriate, if not scientifically absurd, RCTs are for investigating any therapeutic approach, including those that are manualised (Guy *et al.*, 2012). Perhaps much of CBT's popularity is due to how both individually and through the state and other interested parties, psychotherapists attempt to dilute both their own sexuality and potential violence and conspire not to step outside the ideology that contains us all.

In the talking therapies, there was the idea that patients/clients could explore what they found problematic in being clear about themselves. Often, what needed to be spoken about was taboo within the particular culture they came from. However, as a result of the involvement of the state in the talking therapies, there is an increasing possibility that patients/clients cannot now speak of what is not usually permissible or is taboo. There is also the possibility that training does not sufficiently equip talking therapists to hear what is usually not said and for them to be able to stay with not knowing.

One conclusion from the Critical Psychotherapy book (Loewenthal, 2015) is that three very difficult personal and collective courses of action may be required if we are to significantly change our practices: The first is Plato's plea that Therapiea is about continuing to remind ourselves and others that while science and technology are important, they should always come second to the resources of the human soul (Cushman, 2002). Second, we are all capable of good and evil and we therefore need to be aware of those theories that encourage us to sidestep any consideration of our capability for making others wretched. Third, that as individuals we wish to escape through denial unsavoury aspects of ourselves and can therefore be seduced or otherwise forced away from really opening up to both ourselves and our clients/patients. This is facilitated by the powers-that-be, which in our case is neo-liberalist capitalism. Yet the assumption remains that the more we can stay open to all this and work it through, the greater our and others' potential.

There is much to support the idea that the state is using psychotherapy, psychoanalysis and counselling as a form of social control (Hurvitz, 1973). Although it can be argued that oppressing oppresses the oppressor, perhaps it is particularly pertinent that in some ways both oppressors and the oppressed may wish to be oppressed? Perhaps we welcome this 'opportunity'; although both Marx and Nietzsche have suggested in different ways that religion enables people to stop thinking, the demise of religion would appear to have been replaced by the forces of both consumerism and the state, which have resulted in the further development of alienated states of being. For example, state-endorsed therapies tend to either provide a way of directly taking one's mind off what worries one (CBT), or a means of reflecting that we are the person that we would like to think of ourselves as; or, to a decreasing extent, approaches that do neither. What are almost too difficult to find are therapies that allow us to acknowledge the good in ourselves and others without denying our sexuality and violence as well as a place in which we can consider our part in the political set-up.

Perhaps much of what has been written here has already been covered in a different way by Paul Ricoeur (1970) in his 'hermeneutics of suspicion'. Here, rather than we wrongly regard too much as the natural order of things, it is suggested that perhaps it's time we actually see, through Marx and others, how capitalism affects our wellbeing, through Nietzsche how morality is man-made, and through Freud, the secrets of our sexuality. All three notions may give the potential to free ourselves, not completely, but from at least some of that which we didn't even know we were subject to. It is of course understandable that attempts will be made to dismiss Marx, Nietzsche and Freud, again both from the forces in society and those in the individual. I am not suggesting that we shouldn't be critical of them either (we need to be suspicious of their suspicion but not automatically dismissive).

What, if anything, can be done?

So what seems to be clear is that the talking therapies are cultural practices and the ways in which they are researched are also cultural practices. One question is, how do we respond to the inappropriateness of forcing an external empirical research method onto psychotherapy, psychoanalysis and counselling? As Ricoeur (1970) writes, the hermeneutics of suspicion are in opposition to scientific understanding such that, for example, one should not attempt to locate psychoanalysis within the causal discourse of natural sciences. However, qualitative research is often not much of an answer. Although it may help an individual researcher it cannot usually be generalised and indeed shouldn't. Thus the trending notion of practitioner researcher (McLeod, 1999) may mean that, increasingly, trainees are not being best prepared for practice. For example, it may be preferable for these students to consider social, economic and technological contexts or literary studies instead of learning about statistics and a bit of biology. Taking bright people with the desire to help others and filling their minds with substandard technical thinking can be seen as another form of social control. Furthermore, as mentioned, the work of the talking therapist is increasingly becoming detrimental to the therapist's own life as well.

And as for the future training of psychotherapists, could it become more like the training of psychiatrists and psychologists, making those who originally wanted to help others instead be caught up in state-endorsed frameworks.

In concluding my book on critical psychotherapy (Loewenthal, 2015) what emerged for me are two key forces. The first is from the individual who, through what some would call denial, wants to avoid staying with uncomfortable thoughts, fantasies and dreams. The second force is from those in power who do not want those that they manage to understand how this is done.

The concern is that unless psychotherapists can re-establish the place taken by neo-liberalism back to being on the fringes of our society and away from the state, they are rapidly becoming far too much part of the problem rather than the solution.

References

Barber, B. (2000). 'Ballots versus bullets'. *Financial Times*, 20 October 2000.

Barzelay, M. (2001). *The new public management: Improving research and policy dialogue*. Berkeley, CA: University of California Press.

Bentall, R. (2009). Guardian.co.uk [Online]. Available at: www.guardian.co.uk/comment isfree/2009/aug/31/psychiatry-psychosis-schizophrenia-drug-treatments. Accessed 31 August 2009.

Bion, W. R. (1962). *Learning from experience*. London: Heinemann.

Blauner, R. (1964). Alienation and freedom: The factory worker and his industry. *The Sociological Quarterly*, 6(1), 83–5.

Brown, S. & Stenner, P. (2009). *Psychology without foundations: History, philosophy and psychosocial theory*. London: Sage.

Budge, S., Baardseth, T. P., Wampold, B. E. & Flückiger, C. (2010). Researcher allegiance and supportive therapy: Pernicious affects on results of randomized control trials. *European Journal of Counselling and Psychotherapy*, 12(1), 23–39.

Chunn, L. (2013). 'Britain on the couch: UK therapists share our biggest worries', *The Guardian*, 7 December 2013.

Cotton, T. & Loewenthal, D. (2015). Personal versus medical meanings in breakdown, treatment and recovery from 'schizophrenia'. In D. Loewenthal (ed.), *Critical psychotherapy, psychoanalysis and counselling: Implications for practice*. Basingstoke, UK: Palgrave Macmillan.

Cushman, R. (2002). *Therapeia: Plato's Conception of Philosophy*. New Brunswick and London: Transaction Publishers.

Davies, J. (2013). *Cracked: Why psychiatry is doing more harm than good*. London: Icon Books.

Foucault, M. (1971). 'The discourse on language' (trans. Swyre, R.). *Social Science Information*, April, 7–30.

Frie, R. & Orange, D. (eds) (2009). *Beyond postmodernism: New dimensions in clinical theory and practice.* New York: Routledge.

Gruening, G. (2001). Origin and theoretical basis of new public management. *International Public Management Journal*, 4, 1–25.

Guy, A., Loewenthal, D., Thomas, R. & Stephenson, S. (2012). Scrutinising NICE: The impact of the National Institute for Health and Clinical Excellence Guidelines on the provision of counselling and psychotherapy in primary care in the UK. *Psychodynamic Practice*, 18(1), 25–50.

Harding, L. (2014). *The Snowden files: The inside story of the world's most wanted man.* London: Faber & Faber.

Harvey, D. (2007). *A brief history of neoliberalism.* Oxford: Oxford University Press.

Heaton, J. M. (2013). *The talking cure: Wittgenstein on language as bewitchment and clarity.* Basingstoke, UK: Palgrave Macmillan.

Hoffman, I. Z. (2009). Doublethinking our way to 'scientific' legitimacy: The desiccation of the human experience. *Journal of the American Psychoanalytic Association*, 57, 1043–1069.

House, R. & Loewenthal, D. (eds) (2008). *Against and for CBT: Towards a constructive dialogue?* Ross-on-Wye, UK: PCCS Books.

Hurvitz, N. (1973). Psychotherapy as a means of social control. *Journal of Consulting and Clinical Psychology*, 40(2), 232–9.

Lather, P. & St. Pierre, E. A. (2013). Post-qualitative research. *International Journal of Qualitative Studies in Education*, 26(6), 629–33.

Layard, R. (2005). 'Mental health: Britain's biggest social problem?' Paper presented at the No. 10 Strategy Unit Seminar on Mental Health, LSE 20 January 2005. Available at: www.cep.lse.ac.uk/textonly/research/mentalhealth/RL414d.pdf. Accessed: 31 December 2012.

Loewenthal, D. (2010). 'Audit, audit culture and therapeia: Some implications for wellbeing with particular reference to children'. In L. King and C. Moutsou (eds) *Rethinking Audit Cultures: A Critical Look at Evidence Based Practice in Psychotherapy and Beyond*, Ross-on-Wye, UK: PCCS Books, pp. 75–95.

Loewenthal, D. (2011). *Post-existentialism and the psychological therapies: Towards a therapy without foundations.* London: Karnac.

Loewenthal, D. (2014). Are psychological therapists less trustworthy than they used to be? *European Journal of Psychotherapy & Counselling*, 16(2), 97–100.

Loewenthal, D. (ed.) (2015). *Critical psychotherapy, psychoanalysis and counselling: Implications for practice.* Basingstoke, UK: Palgrave Macmillan.

Mace, C., Rowland, N., Evans, C., Schroder, T. & Halstead, J. (2009) Psychotherapy professionals in Europe: Expansion and experiment. *European Journal of Psychotherapy & Counselling*, 11(2), 131–40.

McLeod, J. (1999). *Practitioner research in counselling.* London: Sage.

McNamee, S. (2010). Research as social construction: Transformative inquiry. *Health and Social Change*, 1(1), 9–19.

McNamee, S. (2014). Research as relational practice: Exploring modes of inquiry. In G. Simon & A. Chard (eds), *Systemic inquiry: Innovations in reflexive practice research.* Farnhill, UK: Everything is Connected Press.

Merleau-Ponty, M. (2002[1962]). *Phenomenology of Perception.* London: Routledge.

Middleton, H. (2015). The medical model: What is it, where did it come from and how long has it got? In D. Loewenthal (ed.), *Critical psychotherapy, psychoanalysis and counselling: Implications for practice.* Basingstoke, UK: Palgrave Macmillan.

Miller, J-A. (ed.) (2006). *L'Anti-Livre noir de la psychanalyse.* Paris: Editions du Seuil.

Mollon, P. (2009). The NICE guidelines are misleading, unscientific and potentially impede good psychological care and help. *Psychodynamic Practice*, 15(1), 9–24.

Monbiot, G. (2014). Sick of this market-driven world? You should be. *The Guardian*, 5 August 2014.

Munder, T., Brütsch, O., Leonart, R., Gerger, H. & Barth, J. (2013). Researcher allegiance in psychotherapy outcome research: An overview of reviews. *Clinical Psychology Review*, 33(4), 501–11.

NICE (2009). 'Treatment and management of depression in adults (CG90)'. National Collaborating Centre for Mental Health. Published by The British Psychological Society 2010 [Online]. Available at: www.guidance.nice.org.uk/CG90/Guidance/pdf/English

Parker, I. & Revelli, S. (2008). *Psychoanalytic practice and state regulation*. London: Karnac.

Parry, G., Blackmore, C. Beecroft, C. & Booth, A. (2010). *A systematic review of the efficacy and clinical effectiveness of group analysis and analytic/dynamic group psychotherapy.* Available at: www.academia.edu/2723418/A_systematic_review_of_the_efficacy_and_clinical_effectiveness_of_group_analysis_and_analytic_and_dynamic_group_psychotherapy. Accessed: 17 August 2014.

Pilgrim, D., Rogers, A. & Bentall, R. (2009). The centrality of personal relationships in the creation and amelioration of mental health problems: The current interdisciplinary case. *Health: An Interdisciplinary Journal for the Social Study of Health, Illness and Medicine*, 13(2), 235–54.

Polanyi, M. (1966). *The tacit dimension*. Garden City, NY: Doubleday.

Ricoeur, P. (1970). *Freud and philosophy: An essay on interpretation* (trans. D. Savage). New Haven, CT: Yale University Press.

Rizq, R. (2013). IAPT and thoughtcrime: Language, bureaucracy and the evidence-based regime. *Counselling Psychology Review*, 28(4), 111–15.

Shotter, J. (2005). Inside processes: Transitory understandings, action guiding anticipations, and withness thinking. *International Journal of Action Research*, 1(2), 157–89.

Shotter, J. (2014). Practice-based methods for practitioners in inquiring into the continuous co-emergent 'stuff' of everyday life. In G. Simon & A. Chard (eds), *Systemic inquiry. Innovations in reflexive practitioner research*. London: Everything is Connected Press.

Snell, R. (2007). *L'Anti-Livre Noir de la Psychanalyse*, Jacques-Alain Miller (ed.) Reviewed in *European Journal of Psychotherapy and Counselling*, June, 9(2), 231–39.

Verhaeghe, P. (2014). Neoliberalism has brought out the worst in us. *The Guardian*, 29 September 2014.

Vygotsky, L. S. (1986). *Thought and language*. Cambridge, MA: The Massachusetts Institute of Technology.

3

REGULATION, INSTITUTIONALIZED ETHICS AND THE THERAPEUTIC FRAME

Stuart Morgan-Ayrs

Introduction

In understanding the area to be discussed it is important to briefly consider the historical context. There have been various attempts through the years to introduce regulatory standards and/or registration in the therapy field. This has taken a number of forms, the most visible being the rise of a handful of large professional bodies such as the BACP, UKCP and COSCA, who have attempted, with varying degrees of success, to lay 'claim' to the profession. Most recently the BACP has courted controversy with its move to validate its numerical dominance by applying for a Royal Charter.

Another method of increasing 'market share' has been through the accreditation of qualifications, in both the university and vocational spheres. One such project, which the author was personally directly involved with, involved the adoption of NVQ units and levels for accreditation purposes in complementary and talking therapies, but the project faded away in the late 1990s. National Occupational Standards (NOS), created by 'lead bodies' claiming to represent elements of the professions, have been used as core competencies for many training courses and accreditation routes, but have been widely criticized as being inflexible and unrepresentative of the diversity in the therapeutic field. NOS have, to a varying degree, been adopted as core competencies underpinning voluntary regulation status for many complementary health therapies, but perhaps less so in the psychological therapies where standards remain dominated by the influence of major professional bodies.

Context

Regulation

In recent years two parallel regulatory processes have been under way. Statutory regulation (SR) was frequently proposed for the psychological therapies, while voluntary regulation (VR) remained the Government's preferred choice for the complementary therapies. Confusingly perhaps, hypnotherapy found itself classified as a complementary therapy, despite its obvious psychological nature and close relationship with psychoanalysis. Indeed many integrative therapy training programmes that involve some combination of hypnotherapy with psychoanalysis, analysis, psychotherapy or counselling have followed the VR route, with hypnotherapy as the 'core therapy'.

Ironically herbalism, generally thought of as a complementary therapy, has been scheduled for statutory regulation (SR) instead, creating an interesting anomaly. Statutory regulation (SR), at first for psychologists, and subsequently counselling and psychotherapy, was originally mooted to be handled by an existing regulator, the Health Professions Council, more recently re-branded as the Health and Care Professions Council (HCPC). HCPC took over psychology first, with the dominant British Psychological Society (BPS) acquiescing without so much as a whimper. Indeed there appeared to be a widespread assumption that the change could only bring positive consequences, despite many observers, this author included, wondering why the BPS needed further regulation at all, given it already had Royal Chartered status. A cynic might speculate that further regulation was indeed unnecessary, but the existing status and standards made BPS an 'easy catch' for the HCPC, furthering its long term goal of capturing the psychological therapies.

Psychologists with specific professional titles, working in clinical settings, were captured by the statutory regulation (SR) process, meaning that those titles became protected and subject to statutory regulation (SR). Variations on those titles such as the generic term 'psychologist', 'holistic psychologist', 'positive psychologist', 'analytic psychologist' and so on have not yet been protected or captured by SR and are thus still open to unrestricted use. The capture of psychotherapy and counselling was proposed as the next stage of SR. NOS were not considered appropriate by the HCPC for these professions, so they began to write their own 'standards of competency' to define the profession. Rather than address and rectify those reservations that professionals in the industry had already expressed about the NOS, the HCPC standards began to morph into something even worse and potentially far more draconian and inflexible. A major ideological divide opened up, as the HCPC were attempting to create a narrow reductionist definition of a field that is in reality extremely diverse, flexible and adaptive and, as a matter of principle, is highly resistant to attempts to homogenize its multiplicity of belief systems and standpoints. Alongside this problem of principled resistance, sat a number of major reservations as to the practicality of what was being proposed and, crucially, widespread concern as to whether SR was needed at all. A critical unanswered question was whether SR was actually appropriate at all, and were there other sensible approaches that should have been considered. These questions, along with the lack of due process in considering the alternatives, culminated in a Judicial Review instigated by a number of professional bodies, and this led to criticism of the HCPC's process and a stalling of the regulatory capture process.

Meanwhile voluntary regulation for the complementary therapies had been gathering pace. By 2011 Reflexologists and Hypnotherapists were already being registered with the Complementary and Natural Healthcare Council (CNHC), with other therapies soon to follow, including massage, Shiatsu and forms of acupuncture. Although not without its detractors, including those who continued to question the rationale for its existence, VR was alive and developing fast, while SR was evidently stalling.

The 2010 General Election brought a coalition Government with both the Conservative and Liberal Democrat parties espousing light tough regulation generally, including for the therapy field. The ideology of Labour and its enthusiasm for regulation was replaced with a contrasting mode of thought, leading to the so called 'bonfire of the Quangos'. HCPC and their version of SR was already in place for psychologists, but the new Government brought forward a new proposal, the Accredited Voluntary Register (AVR) scheme. AVR would be maintained by the Professional Standards Agency (PSA), the new name for the Council for Healthcare Regulatory Excellence, the body which already regulated or monitored all the Statutory regulators, including HCPC. AVRs have since been renamed as Accredited Register (AR), dropping the reference to 'voluntary' in order to present a more robust image and brand to the public and professionals alike.

AR was broadly welcomed by the profession, although the cost of achieving AR status was prohibitive for many small professional bodies. As a result many small specialist groups have opted out of the process, others with integrated hypnotherapy plus psychological therapy training have maintained links to the CNHC via the hypnotherapy accreditation route, thus using CNHC as an AR umbrella for their members. Generally, however, the scheme has been a success. Various professional bodies came on board rapidly, including the BACP, UKCP, COSCA and perhaps confusingly CNHC. The Federation of Holistic Therapists (FHT) covering amongst other therapies counselling and hypnotherapy, and the sister bodies the National Hypnotherapy Society and National Counselling Society (NHS & NCS) soon followed. In a relatively short time, compared with the stalling associated with SR, the AR scheme has attracted a high level of support and awareness. A recent development at the time of writing (December 2014), is the PSA revising the accreditation logo to read 'Professional Standards Authority Accredited Register', dropping the word 'voluntary' and emphasising the PSA involvement, arguably implying parity of credibility with SR.

As a footnote to the historical progression, it is worth considering that despite the success of VR and AR to date, there is still pressure to impose SR from a splinter group of labour MPs who insist on linking what they claim is a need for SR with the issue of Conversion Therapy (CT). CT is the widely condemned attempt to use a form of 'therapy' to convert non-heterosexual clients to comply with discriminatory societal heterosexual norms. Prior to AR all the major professional bodies had in any case banned this practice as unethical, and in fact the last bastion of CT followed suit and banned its use in order to gain AR status. AR therefore has already achieved the goal that some claimed would require SR.

For the purpose of this chapter the concept of integrated therapy (IT) is kept as a broad and flexible definition, and refers to any practice involving more than one model of therapy, whether separately (between sessions) or flowing within sessions. SR, via the protection of title, highlights the distinction between roles. Hence clinical psychologists are SR regulated via the HCPC and their job title and role is restricted as such. The same would apply in other statutorily regulated professions such as medical doctors, paramedics and nurses. In order to use a protected title legally, certain qualifications and registrations need to be maintained. In VR or the AR scheme, titles are not directly protected. Therefore, in theory anyone may still call themselves a Counsellor, Psychotherapist or Hypnotherapist. However a VR or AR scheme is not without teeth. The phrase 'accredited counsellor registered with the BACP, a PSA accredited register' could be covered through advertising standards legislation.

Roles and distinctions

So what happens when a therapist uses more than one therapeutic approach? The author works in a busy clinic in Scotland where there are therapists of many types. There are HCPC registered clinical psychologists who provide counselling and sometimes hypnotherapy, there are CNHC registered hypnotherapists also providing counselling, psychotherapy or psychoanalysis, and there are AR scheme registered counsellors and psychotherapists (usually BACP or UKCP) also providing hypnotherapy or forms of psychology. Whether SR or AR or VR registered in a core therapy, the therapists are also providing 'other' forms of therapy in their integrated practice. This may seem obvious to the reader; after all most practitioners complete ongoing professional development leading them to develop other skills and tools over a lifetime of practice, and many deliberately seek out other methods to 'bolt on' or integrate into their professional practice. However when job titles themselves become protected in law, as with statutory regulation (SR), key questions are raised. If the titles 'counsellor' and 'psychotherapist' were to become restricted and subject to SR, for instance, would an HCPC registered psychologist, or a CNHC registered hypnotherapist be able to use them, or practise those therapeutic approaches? Would competent and multiskilled therapists find themselves restricted overnight as to what they could call themselves or offer to clients? Would highly experienced therapists with a recognized core training, and high quality 'bolt on' training in other modalities and skills be forced to 'go back to school' to train again from scratch and achieve legitimate, regulated status separately in each additional therapy? The simple answer is that we do not know, because much would hinge on the precise wording of any regulatory legislation. Unintended and unhelpful consequences could therefore happen quite accidentally!

What are the distinctions that exist in reality between therapy roles? There has been a long term debate in the field for decades as to whether there is a material difference between counselling and psychotherapy, leading to the 'BAC' renaming itself the 'BACP' on the basis of a simple membership vote. Without wishing to take a position on that particular debate, perhaps we can apply similar questioning to other differences? Is psychoanalytic psychotherapy demonstrably different from psychoanalysis? Is analysis (including cognitive behavioural, logical, philosophical etc.) different? Are Lacanian therapists, who use linguistics and discourse, and who might vary their session length, nonetheless providing essentially the same service to a client as Jungians, who use rich symbolism and a strict session length, different? If we dare to contrast the Cognitive Behavioural Therapist (CBT) with an analyst, or a humanistic counsellor with a psychotherapist using analytic or perhaps Cognitive Analytic Therapy (CAT), how can we really know if we are comparing like with like, or looking at completely different phenomena?

Some would say that processes and styles may vary, but essentially all therapeutic relationships are similar, being about the giving of time, space and therapeutic attention to a client for a period of 'professionalized' time. If for a moment we set aside ideological counter arguments, and accept this general premise, we are left with a problem. What, if anything, is the material difference between those therapies which supposedly fall 'outside' the counselling and psychotherapy mainstream and those that for historical or institutional reasons, fall within it? Life coaching essentially uses training and coaching techniques to elicit positive change, but apart from stylistic differences it fits the above broad therapeutic paradigm. Hypnotherapy, now classified by VR as a complementary therapy, also broadly fits the picture, even more so if hypnoanalysis or light trance work including free association is used. In both life coaching and hypnotherapy it is accepted (including in NOS) that verbal discussion prior to the process is necessary to gather information. This is usually carried out in an analytic or counselling style. The reader can doubtless extrapolate many other overlaps and examples of different names for the same basic process. The problem therefore with protecting job descriptions ('protected titles') is this overlap and our inability in practice to define where one therapy begins and another ends.

As well as the potential for well trained and qualified integrative therapists to be prevented from explicitly offering certain therapies that fall outside their 'job title' by name, there is the problem of incentivizing the avoidance of regulation altogether. The more inflexible the process of regulation becomes, the more practitioners will be tempted to avoid it. As already discussed, there are many variations of the 'psychologist' titles that remain completely unprotected. It does not take much imagination to come up with half a dozen unprotected new names for what you do as a therapist, should one want to avoid capture by an SR scheme.

Although I do have criticisms of regulation in any form, it is worth considering that perhaps the AR system can provide the sensible flexibility to enable multiskilled therapists to offer a wide range of services, no matter what their original starting point, training wise. Clinical psychologists leaving NHS practice are able to offer related therapies in which they have trained such as counselling. Hypnotherapists also trained in counselling or analysis can offer those as part of their practice, psychotherapists can offer hypnotherapy having bolted on appropriate training to their core skills. In all cases similar fitness to practise, professionalism, core training and experience tests apply, ensuring the therapist is well qualified, trained and professionally monitored.

Problems of reductionism

Does therapy even need to be broken down into parts in the rather reductionist way favoured by many regulators? For instance, Mindfulness and other Eastern psychological models originated in a culture where religion, philosophy and psychology remained intertwined. The great 'enlightenment' may have had many benefits, but it has encouraged the practice of breaking things down and reducing them to neat, tightly defined categories. Why, I wonder, do we feel the need to do this with therapy at all? Is our profession's apparent obsession with separating and defining therapeutic approaches actually helpful to our clients? Would it make any real difference to clients in practice if we were all called simply 'therapists', for instance? There would be nothing to stop us mentioning that we had particular interests or leanings towards this or that style. We have arguably become trapped in a mode of thinking whereby we must adhere to a strict and narrow definition of certain therapies, or else risk crossing an imaginary line and entering into forbidden professional territory. If I provide a one hour session that includes analysis and some CBT and with the next client I carry out a two hour analysis and hypnosis session, am I changing my very nature as a therapist or just being flexible? Carl Jung pointed out there is only one Jung, and implied we should all get out there and innovate for ourselves. We are perhaps in danger of moving away from the days of innovation and into the realm of self-defeating rigidity and over definition if we allow the regulatory process to dictate what we do, might do, or might think of doing.

The NOS and the proposed HCPC standards share a common danger – the over formalization of the therapeutic conversation. One might argue that, in practice, such standards are a necessary evil, but that in real life no therapist would be willing or even able to comply with dozens of performance criteria while trying to hear what the client is saying; the other possibility though is that the more the standards impinge on the interpersonal process and infiltrate the mind of the practitioner, the more the therapeutic conversation will become highly formulaic and inauthentic. Ackerman and Hilsenroth (2001, p. 171) concluded: 'Therapists' personal attributes such as being rigid, uncertain, critical, distant, tense, and distracted were found to contribute negatively to the alliance'. The possibility of the session being a tick box series of tasks and topics to be covered in such and such a way, takes us so far away from the spontaneous conversation associated with humanistic or most psychoanalytic sessions that the process becomes unrecognizable. Not only does compliance with such externally generated expectations detract from the personal connection and the provision of healing and respectful space, it also calls into question whether the unconscious will be permitted to appear in the session at all. If free association and flowing conversation is required for the unconscious to appear as the 'other' in language, then a stilted procedural approach is unlikely to invite the 'other' into the room. Without that flow there is little opportunity for unconditional positive regard for a humanistic therapist, or for the identification of transference and countertransference for an analyst. We risk cleansing the practice room of the unconscious and removing with it any possibility for meaningful dialogue. Spontaneous expression through movement, analysis of body language and dissonance, identification of defence mechanisms in play, all require time, space and attention. If considering the practice of Lacanian therapy with its unpredictable flexible nature, Jungian therapy with its creativity and symbolism, Eastern psychology with its use of mindfulness, 'being present' and meditation, it is hard to imagine how any of these approaches could fit well with an overly formal structure. In private practice clients often self-refer, looking for a therapy process qualitatively different from the excessively formal and clinical treatment they may have previously received in an NHS or CMHT solution-focused short-term therapy. This is not to undermine the potential usefulness of such services, especially in crisis intervention, but rather to recognize that clients often want to move on to something different, more holistic and dare I say, more relaxed. There is a real danger in over regulation; we might end up failing to provide what is actually needed and wanted by those people we claim to want to assist, the clients themselves.

Part of what might be termed the 'sterilization' of therapy is the removal of its influences. This is ideologically troublesome for those therapists who deliberately study a wide range of schools of thought. The author is reminded of a conversation with a psychotherapy student who reacted with surprise when I mentioned I was studying philosophy of the mind for my latest CPD degree. They had been exposed to a highly sterilized version of psychology, and had no awareness of the study of the mind within philosophy pre-dating the formal 'discovery' of psychology as a scientific discipline. The over formalization of therapy discourages study of related fields like philosophy, theology, symbolism, linguistics, ironically just as the arguably over-sterilized short-term provision of CBT within health services has begun to more explicitly recognize its own philosophical nature and introduce elements of mindfulness. The danger of adopting rigid definitions like those of NOS and SR is that there will be no incentive to learn about what's outside the specific box that is pre-defined for the therapist to live in. In turn the therapists, secure within their sterile box, will only provide a very narrow service to the client. Pope and Keith-Spiegel (2008) conclude that it is in the patient's interests for practitioners, when appropriate, to cross ideological or methodological boundaries on occasion, rather than being constrained within a fixed systematic approach. Therapist professionalism, knowledge and supervision here are the key factors, not sterilization or rigidly defined and audited standards.

Power

There is a danger within any profession that becomes over defined and exact that those who wield 'wisdom' and power within that system come to be considered 'experts'. Consider the respect paid to the General Practitioner medical doctors, who are often expected to know everything about every medical condition by their patients. 'Official advice' sound bites about weight, drinking, exercise, diet and so on are issued as if the doctor is an infallible source of authority. Meanwhile the poor GP is often quite unaware of any contradicting evidence, studies or theories other than those they are expected to peddle on behalf of the hierarchical structure of knowledge embodied by the National Institute for Clinical Excellence (NICE) and the drug companies. If we borrow for a moment the Transactional Analysis model of Parent, Adult and Child: consider that while one is ill one would quite like a nurse or doctor to parent you and make you better, especially if rushed into hospital. Then we can readily understand how the patient can be trapped in a dependent role if the psychological therapy clinic uncritically mirrors that same power dynamic. A paternalistic model of the therapist, analyst or psychiatrist being the fount of all wisdom, the one who interprets and diagnoses, is one we in the psychological therapies tend to consider a historical anachronism. However, if we recreate the old dynamic of expert and patient then we risk reintroducing it by the back door. Add to that power dynamic the widespread use of tests, scores, exercises and tasks often associated with some forms of CBT, and suddenly one is reminded of the image of a child sitting opposite a teacher. Barbanel (1986, p. 82) summarizes the outcomes of the Mays *et al.* (1985) book on negative outcomes in psychotherapy; the primary finding was that 'empathy without training is of limited value and "techniques" without empathy may be the most direct route to negative effects'. Thus over-defined standards may equip one in terms of knowledge, but in terms of application and positive outcomes it is crucial that an appropriate relationship dynamic, which enables true empathy, exists within the therapy room. This removal from the role of 'human equal' is similar to Lacan's theory of psychologists being barred from true understanding of the human mind as a result of being observers seeking the allusive Object 'a' and being dominated by the Body of knowledge (S1) and the master signifiers of knowledge (S2). S1 is underpinned by S2, validating it as scientific 'truth'. Thus the work of the authorities of knowledge underpins what is knowledge, and this defines how one should think about psychology. As Parker (2015, p. 39) observes: 'Students of psychology and subjects of psychological research are treated in such a way that they become disqualified from knowing about themselves, become "embarrassed" about the knowledge they may already have about their own psychology'. If one extrapolates this to the clinic, then if we allow over-definition of therapy by the regulator (who becomes the master signifier S2), thus accepting what regulated therapy is (S1) then this traps us in a paradigm that disbars us from understanding the world of the client.

Agents of our own destruction

Mohr *et al.* (1990, p. 622) concluded about negative outcomes: 'Unfortunately, beyond documenting its presence, very little empirical attention has been brought to bear on the question of whether these negative changes are causally related to psychotherapy or simply incidental observations relating to particularly vulnerable patients.' We have been encouraged to believe that we 'need' regulation and that it is good for us and for clients. We have been fed a narrative in which countless clients will face harm and practitioners will not receive recognition and respect without the supposedly wonderful thing that is regulation. How have we created this myth? Have practitioners come together in an act of Foucauldian subjectifi- cation and created this narrative with all its sources of authority, technologies of the group and technologies of the self? For those not familiar with the idea, Foucault, borrowing from Nietzsche, suggested that groups form themselves, give themselves identity, then create rules for both the group and attitudes that group members have towards themselves. In its original Nietzschian form, the group also requires outside influences to be the 'other' in adversity to the group around which mythology of harm or evil grows. Do we have such 'others'? Are they perhaps the unregulated masses doing evil and harm to patients? Have we fooled ourselves into thinking in this constructed way? Do we need to form such a group and then imagine a wolf outside the door? There is little or no evidence of harm to patients or clients that would be prevented by SR, beyond that already covered by VR, AR or indeed the registration of practitioners with professional bodies generally. If a practitioner were struck off by, for example the UKCP prior to AR, he or she would find it hard to register with another reputable professional body. And those shadier bodies who might accept them would probably still accept them if struck off from a regulated system, simply using a non-regulated job title. Cases involving sexual assault or other criminal behaviour are in all cases a matter for criminal prosecution and thus fall outside the scope of professional regulation. Criminal behaviour is also, self-evidently, not prevented by regulation, as we saw in the Shipman case, and in other recent cases of child molestation by medical personnel. If there really is no evidence that regulation can prevent harm then why have we allowed ourselves to believe it is so urgently needed? Are we perhaps convinced by the narrative that we are somehow second class clinicians compared with regulated practitioners? If we have, then we have obviously forgotten that clients often choose us quite explicitly as a result of the lack of skills and resources offered by the highly regulated, tightly defined and 'professional- ized' NHS.

We appear to be left with a choice between the idea that we have somehow ourselves constructed this narrative through subjectification or, perhaps, other forces have constructed them for us. It has been suggested that the previous Labour Government, who attempted the introduction of SR and who were often criticized as having an appetite for centralization and bureaucracy, had an ideological interest in promoting SR. Could it be that the same Government which provided us with all those CCTV and speed cameras for our own protection were also out to protect us 'for our own good' in the case of the psychological therapies? If this was the case then it appears this was not based on factual evidence of need, but rather on economic vested interests and ideology. The culture of monitor, watch, control that chillingly echoes the grim predictions of Orwell, is not a response to any real risk or need; it is a political response to an unspoken narrative involving power, control and anxiety. Once we uncritically accept and buy into that narrative we become part of it, and take on the mantle of the system. Just as we might be over monitored, watched, controlled and assessed through SR, so the use of imposed standards, systems, assessments and procedures would cascade down into the clinic, so that we too would soon find ourselves controlling rather than enabling clients.

Conclusion

We can also see the influence of other allied bodies in the system of creating and imposing these standards. NICE is a key player in the creation of 'conventional wisdom' for GPs, members of the public and other bodies to consult. NICE appears superficially benign and helpful, but the practical application is notoriously biased towards drug treatment and the use of CBT based psychological therapies. This goes hand in hand with initiatives such as Improved Access to Psychological Therapies (IAPT), supporting and validating the claims that CBT-based therapies are able to provide overarching support for mental health. The powerful triad of drug companies, NICE and IAPT self-validate, leaving patients with the limited recommendations of short-term CBT and/or drugs. Even the language used, such as the job title of 'wellbeing practitioner' by IAPT and 'wellness' generally, together with the Government's obsession with so called 'evidence based' provision creates a paradigm where patients need to be seen to be 'made well', rather than become more self-aware, processing their issues and experiences and moving forward in life. I am not suggesting that there is no place for crisis or short-term intervention in a solution focused way where appropriate; rather I'm asserting that there is no justification for viewing all therapy and client need through a single paradigm, and that to do so may be ultimately destructive of persons and their 'wellness' in the long term. As Woolfolk (2002) points out, there is a need for truth, melancholia and tragedy to be permitted and explored in life. The whole idea of seeking 'wellness' and 'wellbeing' in such an uncritical way seems similar to seeking the Holy Grail, or perhaps a Lacanian object 'a'. If we allow ourselves to be fooled by it then we may sleepwalk into forgetting to do any real therapy work at all.

As a footnote to the idea of CBT-based psychological therapies, it is also ironic, drawing again on the issue of boundaries between therapies and the impossibility of clean distinction, that so many therapies already use what are essentially CBT-based methods. Cognitive Behavioural Coaching, Cognitive Behavioural Hypnotherapy, Mindfulness Based Cognitive Therapy, Cognitive Analytic Therapy and various variations all could be said to offer CBT-based cognitive therapy. So is NICE actually providing any concrete advice when the area is somewhat broad and vague? Again we can see the gap between recommendations or standards and their actual real world implementation. The guidelines from NICE, just like the previous standards from NOS, and the standards originally suggested by HCPC for SR, all give the appearance of specificity, and thus carry the implicit assumption that by defining the scope of practice they will reduce risk and protect the public;

but in practice they are either vague, subjective or, as some argue, unfit for purpose. We return to the key question of regulation itself, if the standards and recommendations are merely lip service, a 'going through of the motions' so as to reassure people and assuage anxiety, how does this actually help support the therapeutic enterprise, for both practitioners and clients? What we see in practice is the creation of distraction and fear, with practitioners scared to cross ill-defined lines, use natural talents or to take even the most justified and appropriate risk. The practitioners are treated by the regulatory system as if they were untrained tabula rasa. Experienced and well trained professionals should have a good idea how to proceed with a case without reference to abstract regulations, especially if they are receiving effective clinical supervision. Imposed SR standards treat practitioners as incompetents who cannot be trusted with the patient's 'wellbeing', while simultaneously 'dumbing down' the profession.

In approaching a conclusion it should be noted that all is not bleak. The accredited Register and VR have permitted far more variety and diversity than SR, and as long as SR is resisted then client choice will remain. Should AR become too restrictive, then practitioners will be able to vote with their feet and leave such schemes since they are voluntary. Thus it is in the mutual self-interest of registers and practitioners to cooperate to make the system as inclusive and diverse as possible. The two main dangers are both likely results of any future imposition of SR. The first as discussed is a fragmentation of integrated therapy through the introduction of artificial divisions between types of therapy. The second is the issue of creeping standardization, going against the needs of clients and dumbing down therapy as we know it. How do we prevent such fragmentation and standardization? First, the profession can come together to support the compromise of the AR schemes so as to make the system increasingly robust, thus rendering SR redundant in the field. Second, principled non-compliance, as used by some teachers who simply refused to mark spurious tests of children, could be instigated en masse in the psychological therapies if SR were to be attempted again. This would essentially make it more difficult for a Government to impose SR than to seek a workable compromise. Third, the least palatable option, in the event of SR, to simply re-name our work and carry on, turning the narrow proscriptive nature of title based regulation back against itself. This last option would be a sad outcome since, as many have commented, we therapists surely own our job titles, not the Government.

When one has trained, qualified and practised as a psychotherapist or counsellor, there is something chillingly Orwellian and intrusive about having the right to that identity threatened by Government decree. Above all, therapists need to keep alive a critical discourse around the psychological therapies and their place in society, and continue to be robust in asserting that not only is there no evidence to support the introduction of SR but also that on the balance of probabilities, its imposition would do far more harm than good. As a profession we have already refused to 'go quietly into the night' as our counterparts in branches of psychology seemed to under the HCPC, and we will need to foster and maintain that spirit of questioning, debate and, if necessary, resistance, in the years ahead.

The work of the Alliance of Counselling and Psychotherapy (2015), together with other allied organisations and politicians have together encouraged the introduction of the workable and rational compromise of AR into the field of the psychological therapies. There is still a clear and present danger of SR being resurrected, with all the associated possibilities for damage to provision, diversity and standards. It is vital that those who value the psychological and complementary therapies remain alert, informed and actively involved in the future of what is our (and not the Government's) profession.

References

Ackerman, S. J. & Hilsenroth, M. J. (2001). A review of therapist characteristics and techniques negatively impacting the therapeutic alliance. *Psychotherapy: Theory, Research, Practice, Training, 38*(2), 171–85. doi:10.1037/0033–3204.38.2.171.

Alliance For Counselling and Psychotherapy (2015). Downloaded in 2015 from: www.allianceforcandp.org/.

Barbanel, L. (1986). Review of 'Negative outcome in psychotherapy and what to do about it'. *Psychotherapy: Theory, Research, Practice, Training, 23*(1), 182–3. doi:10.1037/h0085587.

Mohr, D. C., Beutler, L. E., Engle, D., Shoham-Salomon, V., Bergan, J., Kaszniak, A. W. & Yost, E. B. (1990). Identification of patients at risk for nonresponse and negative outcome in psychotherapy. *Journal of Consulting and Clinical Psychology, 58*(5), 622–8. doi:10.1037/0022-006X.58.5.622.

Parker, I. (2015). *Psychology after Lacan. Connecting the clinic and research. Psychology after Critique.* Abingdon/New York: Routledge Press.

Pope, K. S. & Keith-Spiegel, P. (2008). A practical approach to boundaries in psychotherapy: Making decisions, bypassing blunders, and mending fences. *Journal of Clinical Psychology, 64*(5), 638–52. doi:10.1002/jclp.20477.

Woolfolk, R. L. (2002). The power of negative thinking: Truth, melancholia, and the tragic sense of life. *Journal of Theoretical and Philosophical Psychology, 22*(1), 19–27. doi:10.1037/h0091192.

4

MANAGED MENTAL HEALTHCARE IN THE USA AND THE CARE OF THE SOUL

William Bento

Introduction

The opinions concerning managed mental health care range from praise to blame. The praise is rarely about a qualitative improvement in mental health care services and treatment for the client, but about the administrative efficiency and financial savings for insurance companies. Yet, critical commentary is on the rise on many fronts, including allegations that it could adversely affect quality of care, access to care, the therapist/client relationship, the client's freedom to receive the treatment desired and limited informed patient choice. Given the heterogeneity among managed mental health care organizations throughout the United States – each with differing demographics, stated aims of service and philosophical orientations – it is difficult to evaluate the therapeutic, ethical and community impact of each organization. In this chapter I will identify and examine the many layered concerns about managed mental health care concentrating on the problems that are unique to managed mental health care and how they affect the field of psychotherapeutic practice. This examination will be undertaken by viewing the societal institutional context in which mental health managed care is embedded, the moral/ethical dimensions that arise from such implementation, and the nature of the mental health paradigm as it applies to the care of the soul.

Taking objection to managed mental health care

The term managed health care does not necessarily conjure up an image of a healthy robust human being. The term itself is an extension of the prevailing world outlook that implies all things on earth, inclusive of human beings, can be effectively managed as objects as long as we define our objectives. The faulty premise here is natural science has proven all matters can be subjected to the power of the intellect's capacity to analyse, organize and devise alternative ways of functioning. Yet, the reality is that after over 150 years of utilizing the natural scientific method it has only created more ecological problems than it has managed to solve. The ecological dangers now facing humanity have not diminished but have escalated. To paraphrase Albert Einstein, 'You cannot expect to solve problems with the same type of thinking that caused the problem in the first place'. I conjecture to say the same is true for our mental health issues. Despite the advances and proponents of the managed mental health care systems our national average of mental health is no greater than it was at the outset of managed mental health care.

Spurred by the enactment of the U.S. Health Maintenance Organization Act of 1973, managed care for mental health services has now become a predominant feature in the United States. Proponents and critics have been sharply divided on the impact and effectiveness of the quality of care it has upon mental health services. Proponents, health maintenance organizations (HMOs) take the view that it will benefit patients, providers, payers and society. Critics have voiced their objections to the trend of managed mental health services claiming it will limit patients' choice of providers and treatments, as well as reducing quality of and access to care. Another one of their objections is that the system is set up to disrupt the caretaker and patient relationship. By putting a limit to the number of sessions allowed for a specific diagnostic mental illness not only is the therapeutic process potentially disrupted, the whole idea of treating a person is replaced with the idea of an equation for a diagnostic illness. This disregards the level of severity of the mental health condition and the sanctity of the doctor–patient relationship. These considerations are often overlooked or minimized on the basis that the managed care system is designed to meet the needs of many who are unable to pay fee-for-services or for those whose health care benefits are negligible (Heam, 1994). An added argument for the proponents of managed care for mental health services is the services are frequently unneeded or provided inefficiently and, if not marginally beneficial, perhaps even cause further illness (England & Vaccaro, 1991).

It may be worthwhile to provide a historical background to the leverage managed care has amassed. Due to the unprecedented, and at times unwarranted, expansion of mental health services in the 1980s and the lack of regulation, profiteers entered the market. In particular inpatient drug and alcohol abuse treatment programmes and adolescent psychiatric programmes grew exponentially. Misuse and abuse of these programmes gave the proponents of managed care for mental health a rationale for a political and economic takeover of mental health services (Jellinek & Nurcombe, 1993). The down side to this self-righteous authority lives on in the imposed limitation to treatment for substance abuse and inpatient acute care in general. As these sanctions continue the rate of substance abuse continues to sky rocket. Why? Because drug and alcohol abuse counsellors have been sidelined by the decision-makers, who have assumed how long the course of treatment should take (Harbin, 1994). This is indeed a sad indictment of managed care for mental health. Administrative decisions and policies governing services are for the most part focused on economic efficiency and not on the severity of the addiction. The techniques employed by the advocates of managed care include rejecting elective outpatient care and limiting inpatient days, increasing co–payments for outpatient visits, establishing gatekeepers, using non-psychiatrists for mental health care other than medication management, and requiring specialized utilization review. The new attempts to manage mental health care simply continue practices found in fee-for-service medicine.

Opponents of the managed mental health care have good reason to be concerned. Historically, 'mental health services have long been the neglected step-child of health services'. With the increased management of mental health services, the long-standing discriminatory policies that tend to not cover mental illness and/or to pay only the bare minimum in many instances is bound to grow. With the economic hardships of these times, conventional health insurance plans and HMOs are restricting mental health benefits more stringently than they do medical care benefits. The upshot of this situation is that it is a standard that HMOs are setting caps on services – numbers of hospital days or outpatient visits or by imposing limits on the annual or lifetime dollars that support for mental health services can receive (Grob, 1991). Scandals by administrators of mental health services and widely publicized exploiters of the mental health service organizations, such as homeless persons with mental illness, cast a dark shadow on the services provided to the mentally ill. As a result of this and the deep-seated convictions that the mentally ill are often perceived to be the cause of their own problems, benefits and generous funds normally given to medical problems are limited or denied to advocates for mental health. The unfortunate bias that sees the nature of mental illness as a dichotomy between mind and body tends to minimize the physical and mental suffering and disability associated with mental illness as compared with that of someone who has lost a limb or someone who is struggling with heart disease or a bout with cancer, for instance.

Although it may seem ludicrous to question the value of psychotherapy in a time where it is well established in the public domain, it is still a hotly debated subject among professionals in the medical and mental health field. The relative lack of proof of the effectiveness of mental health treatment based on psychotherapy remains a major roadblock in the further development of mental health services. The notion that psychotherapy is designed for the intellectually endowed and privileged wealthy fosters the idea that it is a luxury and not a necessity for mental health. Along with this opinion is the misinformed idea that mental health care is typically a lengthy and expensive proposition. In the absence of empirical and convincing research it is challenging to distinguish effective and established psychotherapies and interventions from the latest fads (Wells & Brooks, 1989). The lack of consensus among the mental health professionals about effective psychotherapy has given the medical/psycho-pharmacological interventions precedence for insurance companies and HMOs. I have a number of concerns about this.

Concern number 1

Proponents of the anti-managed mental health care are concerned that the growing trend to measure a successful mental health service by the dollars saved and the treatment time decreased will only result in less costly providers and treatments and less intensity or quantity of service. The quality of treatment is likely to be sacrificed by the non-psychiatric mental health decision-makers who are often unaware of or insufficiently trained or unconcerned about the effect of their decisions on the quality of treatment. The tendency to rely on outcomes data and practice guidelines designed to economically manage mental health care services all but eclipses any true and holistic evaluation on the quality of care. There is yet to be any conclusive research establishing the fact that using data driven methods improves the quality of care (McCarthy, Gelber & Dugger, 1993).

Defining the acceptable quality of care has not yet reached a global consensus. There is no agreed-upon level of care that has been regarded as the standard. Preliminary research evidence found in *Focus*: June 1993 in an article entitled 'Data Show Mixed Results for Managed Care' suggests that quality of care in fee-for-service mental health care is similar to that in managed mental health care. Before we can come to a determination of the acceptable quality of care in mental health services we must be clear not to confuse it with quantity of care. Contrary to popular opinion, more services do not always equate to better outcomes and higher degree of satisfaction. However, there exists among HMOs the justification that fewer services can safeguard the escalating costs derived from undesirable medical, psychological and social consequences from too many unnecessary services. This rationale gains support in the absence of a good and acceptable definition of quality (Boyle & Callahan, 1993).

Concern number 2

A secondary concern beyond that of quality is the concern of access to services. The claim of managed care services is that it enhances access to care and does so in a more timely and appropriate manner than financially restrictive, traditional fee-for-services. However, one often overlooked aspect is that even managed care has co–payments, particularly in outpatient mental health services. The more service one needs the more the co-payments rise.

The confounding problem in collecting reliable data for ascertaining there is greater access through managed care is that many persons with mental illness do not seek out services for a multitude of understandable reasons – the tendency to cover up mental illness, the stigma of shame or being perceived as having a deficiency, the set of priorities that devalues a sense of wellness, the expectation that the cost is not worth it and so on. Hence, there is no empirical evidence that managed care is preferable to fee-for-services. There are too many variances to HMOs' costs for varying vendor services, varying benefit packages and in varying demographic areas to extract reasonable data that would apply to all. The variables at play in the question of limiting access on the part of policy makers in managed care is in itself a costly endeavour. Assessing the severity of symptoms and the failure of previous treatments to establish protocols and a list of mental health practitioners to be placed on an approved referral list is time consuming and makes the entry into accessible mental health care a bureaucratic affair.

Concern number 3

The impact of managed mental health care upon the patient/provider relationship has both short and long-term effects. In both cases the effect is adverse. There is no way that it can be considered an improvement upon the fee-for-services model. It is an additional complication on what has always been a very subjective matter. Mental health practitioners and psychotherapists are bound to be less invested in the course of treatment as long as they are faced with the continual prospect of being governed by the HMO as to what they can and cannot do, how long they can work with the patient and when they can expect to receive their payment for services delivered. Added to this complication is the dilemma of being required to disclose sensitive and confidential patient information to managed mental health care organizations to obtain approvals for treatment. And lastly, there is the threat to the continuity of care when the gatekeepers direct patients to preferred mental health professionals. Patients may be persuaded to change to exclusively credentialed and approved providers of the HMO. Patients may also face the dictum that they may only see a psychiatrist if prescription drugs are warranted or when their conditions require hospitalization (Jellinek & Nurcombe, 1993). It is not merely policies excluding and redirecting services that come into question here. It is also the methods of persuasion that need examination, for many of them are coercive in limiting care. Providers once had an unencumbered pathway of making decisions for more or less care. Their autonomy and authority was unquestionable. With managed mental health care that is no longer the case. HMOs are customarily offering providers financial incentives to provide less care – such as end of the year bonuses or pay increases for services. This practice places the providers' financial gain above the patients' best interests, which has traditionally been considered the therapists' primary obligation.

Along with the ethical dilemma of being required to disclose patient information to the mental health organization to meet criteria and approval for care, there is the delicate moral imperative that only those who have legitimate reason to work with the information be given access to it. In the case of mental health the risk of damage and stigmatization is greater when private information is circulated out of indiscretion. Herein lies the thorny thicket of therapeutic and ethical concerns.

Unless the agency of HMOs can carry an equal commitment with the providers for the sacredness of the patient/provider relationship, interruptions in the flow of treatment will continue to challenge the integrity of all involved. It is well known that the initial therapeutic bond is the most potent means for effective treatment of mental illnesses.

Concern number 4

Managed mental health care organizations are run as businesses that provide services. Like all businesses there is a competitive drive to stay pertinent, vital and to promote their service as the best in the marketplace. Healthcare and the marketplace make strange bedfellows. One of the most common casualties in this arena is the truth. The need for education accompanies the need to make informed choices. How are HMOs doing at the point of enrolling and at the point of offering their services to a population that is often impaired in their capacity to assess the pros and cons of decision-making? Do they disseminate the full scope and limit of benefits to their prospective client? Are they forthcoming about what services are not in their plan and where such services may be made available? It is difficult enough for the average employee to decide which heath plan is suitable for him and his family. Not all persons have a choice in such health plans. And even when there is a choice it is not always understood how a chosen plan limits or provides access to care and what the health consequences of the limits may be. For a person with mental illness, who is often in denial of his or her condition, understanding their rights, privileges and limitations to care is a greater issue. And greater still when their judgment is impaired by their mental illness. This issue demands that the managed mental health care provider must take this into consideration or be culpable of exploiting their client.

Concern number 5

Given the above consideration of the problematic issues of informed patient choice in the mental health field, it is not hard to see that many HMO benefit packages are designed in a capricious and unfair manner. For a long time many mental health service organizations created health care plans in which their decision protocols and criteria for a network of mental health services were not transparent. Although there is a change in this area and in the methods of appeal for uncovering arbitrary policies impacting a person's right to service, the hidden agenda set out at the beginning of the HMOs still impacts the field. There is no parity between mental health and general health benefits. It is difficult to morally justify the non-parity of these benefits, but the long-standing devaluation of persons with mental disabilities remains prevalent. It is less evident in the benefit designs that give greater preference to biologically based mental illness.

Evidence-based research needs to gather around the effectiveness of non-medical treatments, such as intensive care management, residential care facilities and the multidisciplinary approaches and services for mental illness, and the modified training and work programmes designed to give the mentally challenged person a stake in a meaningful role in society (Boyle & Callahan, 1993). It is this disparity between the medical science oriented approach and the humanistic/holistic views found in psychological and sociological paradigms that underlie the divide. The research to support the former is quantitative and considered empirical, whereas the latter research is qualitative and phenomenological. These two approaches need not be seen as incompatible, but should be understood as valid perspectives to seeing the whole.

Lastly, this problem of bringing balanced views into understanding the impact of managed mental health care will require an objective oversight of how the decision-making procedures are influenced by biases. One particular bias concerns the terms 'medical necessity and medically effective', which seem to carry scientific weight in terms of credibility. The terms are ambiguous and are often linked to interpretations that are loaded with bias. The balancing solution to this issue is to invite all players in mental health to the table (patients, families, health care professionals and the managed health organization representatives). It is these individuals who need to open up the public dialogue before the health care policies become cast-iron policies. The creation of a representative consumer/provider panel can contribute to the development of greater parity and more open and inclusive decision processes providing effective mental health services.

Concern number 6

There is little doubt that managed mental health care has moved decision-making away from the patient – first by co-opting his mental health care needs into a system of management and second, by diminishing the mental health care provider's capacity to deliver services. The wizard behind the curtain here is not as often held responsible for the outcome of health care services – that is, the health care manager or utilization reviewer. There is a shift in responsibility that needs to be recognized. It has two major moral challenges to it.

1   The uneven split of power and responsibility between the manager of mental health and the provider of the therapies. If the course of development for managed care is that the manager of mental health services continues to assume authority over the treatment planning, it must be willing to bear the burden of responsibility for its outcome. If the course forward can turn to a shared responsibility, then the patient or family, manager and provider must come to terms in defining the legal and clinical lines of accountability

2   There is a need to re-examine the public debate about the proponents and the critics of managed mental health care. The debate has been polarized into a 'for or against' managed care position. The focus completely ignored the social fabric in which the patient and provider are embedded. The core issue is fundamentally a moral and philosophical one. The question of what does access to care mean and the standard to what is reasonable care for safe-guarding mental health is hardly discussed. These questions cannot be adequately addressed with the dominant worldview of materialism in mind, for it is an infectious illness contaminating our thinking, our feeling and what we are creating in terms of mental illness. The ironic situation is that we are caught in the web of iatrogenics, that is, our solution for advancing better mental health care is in fact creating greater problems. To reiterate what was stated earlier in paraphrasing Albert Einstein, 'You cannot expect to solve problems with the same type of thinking that caused the problem in the first place'.

A commentary on the concerns about managed mental health care: deeper considerations

From the lens of a Transpersonal Psychologist and Anthroposophic Psychotherapist, there are four key areas of this debate worth expounding upon. Forgive me if I become aphoristic in my commentary, but these issues are far too large to explicate in a brief chapter of a book. Nevertheless, I do hope to offer a few salient ideas to the way this debate can be understood – more from the absence of ideas than from a criticism of its current formulation.

The term we use with psychological imbalances is mental illness, but we all know it refers to much more than a mental problem. It involves emotional dysregulation and an inability to control one's own will, alongside a disturbance in perception and processing of ideas. Yet, rather than addressing the whole imbalance of thoughts, feelings and behaviours we have adopted a short hand view of it and lumped it into the term mental illness. Unfortunately, when Sigmund Freud was translated into English his term 'psyche' was interpreted to mean mind or mental apparatus, where in fact he meant the soul – a much broader concept than the mind. One of the most distinctive factors in Transpersonal Psychology is its recognition that a redemption of the word psyche needs to be boldly declared. The soul is the realm wherein our interior life unfolds. And it is this realm that we experience, and that determines the quality of our life.

I am convinced if we were courageous enough to talk about mental illness as soul imbalances and to advocate for mental health being a wholesome approach to soul care, we would re-envision how we would proceed with matters of health and illness.

Key area 1

The illusion with managed care is that it fosters a tendency to abdicate vital decisions and activities of self-care. Such programmes as managed care only solidify the general notion that 'doctors know best'. As a result authority is transferred from the patient to the representative of the system of managed care, which is not always the doctor but may be the gatekeeper of MHO policies. It is a by-product of managed care. So in effect, the decisions for the soul care of the mental health patient are being taken by people who do not have a relationship with the patient nor a true understanding of the prognosis and the type of treatment being administered. So in the end a script is being given to the provider that is based on a diagnosis and not an understanding of an individual. For instance, a major depression may be treated by limiting it to ten sessions and supplementing with anti-depressant medications regardless of the wishes of both provider and patient. The insidious nature of managed care is the subtle forms of dependency and learned helplessness it creates. Managed care practices tend to undermine the 'I' that, in an anthroposophical practice, is the key factor for taking responsibility for one's health and welfare. The 'I' must be actively engaged in the process of treatment. This is not well understood. As it is now, the guiding idea of managed care is not so different from that of maintaining an efficient machine. The analogy is intentional. By default, the language used to speak about the maladies of dysfunction to a human being is mechanistic. The healing paradigm for mental illnesses are captured in phrases such as, 'he has a missing screw', 'she is not running on all four cylinders', 'he has his wires crossed', as if the person has broken parts that need to be fixed or replaced. It is this type of careless thinking that strips the human being of his dignity.

Key area 2

Managed care of mental health, by its very nature, seeks to not only manage the care, it seeks to control who is qualified to be a managed care practitioner and what forms of psychotherapy are sanctioned and what are not. A practitioner such as myself, who practises out of a spiritual orientation, finds it difficult to get by the gatekeepers of the HMO even though I am qualified with the appropriate credentials and licence. This forces the provider and the patient into moral dilemmas in the documentation for approval to administer care and in how one assigns diagnosis for billable services. It also limits the practitioner's capacity to utilize the full array of resources in the course of treatment. Scripted care protocols limit the creative and innovative capacity of the clinician or therapist. Furthermore, it may curtail collaborative and transdisciplinary approaches as well as accessing community support resources often utilized in progressive treatment approaches.

Key area 3

Due to the prevailing model of psychopathology, managed care is often focused on the severity of mental illnesses at the expense of some of the more commonplace disturbances and soul imbalances such as adjustment disorders or personality disorders. The HMOs also overlook the basic necessities of proactive maintenance of mental health care. Without providing education about healthy lifestyles, the chronic relapse into patterns of behaviour that set up soul imbalances will continue. This absence of proactive and preventative care unwittingly supports chronic mental illness. The reliance placed on psycho-pharmacological interventions slants most educational aspects of managed mental health care to the rationale for medication and the necessity for compliance. Rarely will you find an HMO providing information on alternatives or addressing the pros and cons of the psychiatric medications.

Key area 4

Misconceptions of psychotherapy and outright rejection of psychotherapy as 'unscientific' are unjustified. These views, which cast a long shadow on psychotherapy, arise from a narrow scientism rather than from sound principles of the philosophy of science (Holmes & Lindley, 1989). The adoption of the view that psychotherapy is simply a diversion or a luxury plays far too great a role in HMO policies, where, in fact, it should be like education and understood as an essential component to health care in a post-modern society. One of the most persistent concerns in giving credibility to psychotherapy is the possibility that any good outcome may be perceived as not the result of psychotherapeutic theory or effective technique, but of the personal influence the therapist has over the patient. Rather than seeing it as a matter of control or influence, it could be seen as the expertise of the psychotherapist in establishing a trusting rapport that engages and empowers the patient to take hold of his or her soul forces. Yet, the prevalent view is bound up with bio-medical interventions. If psychotherapy involved evaluation of a drug, its effectiveness would be relatively straightforward.

Modern psycho-pharmacology rests on the scientific verification of matching a drug to a disease, whereas psychotherapy depends on the establishment of a relationship between people, which may take precedence over both the technique of a therapist and the ailment of the patient. Unlike drug therapy, psychotherapy consists of a combination of general or non-specific features such as interest, compassion and reliability, together with particular therapeutic interventions ranging from removing cognitive distortions, exploring emotional triggers, changing behaviours and so on. If managed care would give more value to psychotherapy and stop taking a stance that dismisses it as unscientific or too costly, more genuine soul care that strikes at the core of soul imbalances could be offered. And the disturbing issue of denying or interrupting psychotherapy could be eliminated from managed mental health care services. Although this sounds idealistic and naive it is only one step in the right direction. A great deal of research needs to be done to convince the scientific community of psychotherapy's validity. And lastly a more assertive and vigorous dialogue must be dedicated to dismantling the prevailing scientific materialistic view of the human being. We must reclaim the dignity of the human soul when dealing with questions of health and illness.

What if . . .

What if the managed mental health care system was to diminish their interest in psychopathology and increase their interest in salutogenesis; that is to say, addressing the client's potential for health as opposed to illness? What if the norm for providing services was based on the image of the ideal healthy human being rather than the dysfunctional broken person? Does it not make sense that providers make their decisions for mental health care based on the prognosis of what the ideal functioning of that specific person could be rather than fixate on the diagnosis of the person's illness? If our starting point for providing services is the way we think, then it becomes obvious that if we see the person as a carrier of psychopathology we set ourselves up to treat the symptoms related to the disorder. But if we see the person as a developing human in a struggle to overcome deficiencies or impediments, we are compelled to find opportunities for strengthening and guiding the person to find healthy ways of living.

References

Boyle, P. J. & Callahan, D. (1993). Minds and hearts: Priorities in mental health services. *Hastings Center Report* (September–October): S3–S23.

England, M. J. & Vaccaro, V. A. (1991). New systems to manage mental health care. *Health Affairs* (Winter): 129–37.

Grob, G. (1991). *From asylum to community: Mental health policy in modern America*. Princeton, NJ: Princeton University Press.

Harbin, H. T. (1994). Inpatient services: The managed care view. In R. Schreter, S. Sharfstein & C. Schreter (eds), *Allies and adversaries: The impact of managed care on mental health services* (pp. 1–30). Washington, DC: American Psychiatric Press.

Heam, W. (1994). Managing Medicaid. *American Medical News* (19 December): 15–19.

Holmes, J. & Lindley, R. (1989). *The values of psychotherapy*. Oxford: Oxford University Press.

Jellinek, M. S. & Nurcombe, B. (1993). Two wrongs don't make a right: Managed care mental health and the marketplace. *Journal of the American Medical Association* (13 October): 1737–1739.

McCarthy, P., Gelber, G. & Dugger, D. (1993). Outcome measurement to outcome management: The critical step. *Administration and Policy in Mental Health* (September): 59–68.

Wells, K. & Brooks, R. (1989). The quality of mental health services: Past, present and future. In C. Taube, D. Mechanic & A. Homann (eds), *The future of mental health services research* (pp. 203–24). Washington, DC: National Institute of Mental Health.

PART II

Mainly IAPT

5

CONTAINING ANXIETY IN SOCIAL CARE SYSTEMS AND NEO-LIBERAL MANAGEMENT DOGMA

Ian Simpson

> Government by the people for the people becomes meaningless unless it includes major economic decision-making by the people for the people. This is not simply an economic matter. In essence it is an ethical and moral question, for whoever takes the important economic decisions in society ipso facto determines the social priorities of that society.
>
> *Jimmy Reid (1972)*

Introduction

'Learned helplessness', 'long-term emotional abuse', 'attempt to find technocratic perfection', 'permanent and constant change', 'conveyor belt medicine', 'industrialised healthcare', 'centralised control and command culture', 'commodified care', 'patients not profits'. . . . These are some of the comments from a large group of healthcare clinicians who attended the second of a series of meetings aimed at Creating a Healthier NHS which took place in November 2014. They reflect the feelings of anger, disenchantment, demoralisation and dissatisfaction expressed about the current condition of the NHS in the United Kingdom at this time and about recent politically directed changes which have been occurring. A political movement for change is forming to lobby for a different culture in health and social care. Although the desire for change is undoubtedly political, it is given added validity and credence because it is informed by the personal clinical experiences of those actively involved.

For many years now the culture of the NHS has been eroded and fundamentally altered by economic and political changes and developments that have created a traumatised organisation which, as hard as it may try, can no longer uphold the aims and ideals around which it was formed. This is about the destruction of a model. A contextual and collectivist model which, in my view, is demonstrably essential to all aspects of social care. The NHS was created by the ideal that good healthcare should be available to all, regardless of wealth – a social care system which aims to create a healthier and more equitable and harmonious society overall. This is based on three core principles. It should meet the needs of everyone, should be free at the point of delivery and should be based on clinical need, not the ability to pay. These principles are enshrined in the ethos of the NHS but they are being decimated by the neo-liberal business model (New Public Management) currently being advocated by politicians and NHS managers. This represents the vested interests and values of an elite establishment, which prizes individual interest and enterprise over collective cooperation and social cohesion. The expansion of private healthcare creaming off the most profitable services, the 'personalised' care agenda, the Private Finance Initiatives and the primacy of politically directed, 'evidence-based' short-term clinical treatment models are the all too prevalent examples of this development. In the words of Dr John Lister, the journalist and health campaigner:

> A pernicious epidemic is stalking the health care systems of the world. It is striking rich and poor alike, with understandably the most devastating impact on the poorest. It saps vital resources, dislocates and fragments systems, obstructs the development of equitable healthcare systems, and prevents government planning and responding to health needs.
>
> The epidemic is not a medical problem, but a man-made disaster. It is the rampant spread of neo-liberal, pro-market 'reforms', devised and promoted by a narrow policy-making academic and political elite in the wealthiest countries. It can only be eradicated by the spread of information, political campaigning and critical thinking, with regular injections of evidence and social solidarity.
>
> *(Lister, 2013)*

Although neo-liberal economic theory purports to promote equality through unfettered free enterprise, this is based upon a false premise. We are not 'all in it together'. The inequality between the 'haves' and the 'have-nots' means that everyone does not start from the same position. In fact, many eminent economists, including leaders at the IMF and World Bank, now recognise that increasing inequality has serious adverse consequences for the productivity, well-being and effectiveness of any society. This is now being recognised as a major challenge for the future (Dobson, 2007; Stieglitz, 2012; Krugman, 2012: Piketty, 2014; Wilkinson & Pickett, 2009). Similarly, the elevation of individual acquisition and advantage above social need does not provide us with a secure enough foundation for social care systems.

In this chapter, I will explore the consequences of the attempt to impose this contextual model upon one which, in my view, was effectively and efficiently serving the needs of the staff who worked in the service and the patients they cared for. The model we were working with, is, I believe, a prerequisite for the establishment of any social care system and is based upon a bio–psycho–social understanding of human relationships. This includes the importance of a safe enough, actively supportive and containing context for staff and service users, which allows for flexibility, creativity and dialogue when considering treatment models, working relationships and organisational dynamics. Following on from the work now emerging in neuroscience on early infant/caregiver interactions, showing how these provide the basic stepping stones which enable us to move into the extended world of family and social relations, we should expand this into the wider social context of the workplace, optimally establishing a creative, empathic, developmental understanding of the relational interactions between the organisation, the staff and the patients to form secure, healthy, reciprocally beneficial, co-regulated patterns of behaviour.

The psychotherapy service we developed over 25 years began as a small department with one consultant medical psychotherapist, helped by a small group of part-timers. Over the years we managed to expand and grow the service to one in which there were 20 whole time equivalent paid staff with 70 honorary trainees on weekly placement. The service offered a variety of treatment models, including long- and short-term individual psychotherapy, group psychotherapy, training, consultation and reflective practice facilitation to other mental health services, both inside and outside the wider organisation. In 2012 we were confronted by what was called a 'reconfiguration' process (a euphemism for service cuts of over 70 per cent). When this occurred we were seeing over 300 patients each week. Of course, like any reasonably sized service with a hierarchical pay and status structure in place and the inevitable professional and personal dynamics colliding as they do, we were far from perfect. However, we were able to deal with and contain these at a manageable level because of the sense we had of the basic requirements needed to underpin and stabilise our working model. This was based upon a set of holding principles formed by an analytic and thoughtful holistic understanding, reflective spaces for staff, which facilitated thinking and working through issues and difficulties and, most importantly, the maintenance of a safe enough/good enough context as a container that will hold staff and patients together throughout these processes.

As our service developed, we were informed by our training and professional practice, which enabled us to move towards an understanding, reinforced by experience, that containment and holding staff and patients was a group/social phenomenon, embedded in our interrelatedness and connectedness rather than one which focused solely or primarily on individual psychopathology.

These principles, which I believe, are fundamental for social care systems, have, for some time now, been actively undermined by the business/targets and performance model (NPM) which aims to develop and establish neo-liberal market reforms in social care (Griffiths, 1983; Hood, 1991; DoH, 2007). This holds great sway with politicians and the current NHS management. In the attempt to maintain relational security and individual and organisational containment, the business/performance model, in my view, actively deconstructs these principles

---

BOX 1 Containment

Containment is a term often used but not always understood. It refers to the process of psychologically 'holding' an individual or a group of people who fear that their feelings are spiralling out of control and could overwhelm not only them but also those close to them, personally or professionally. It cannot be achieved by offering bland reassurances. Rather, it requires actively offering an understanding of what is happening and demonstrating that a person's anxiety or distress is not necessarily overwhelming but can be addressed and managed. Setting limits, maintaining boundaries and not attempting to unnecessarily suppress their distress is an essential part of the process. It is important to 'stay with' the person or the group in distress and work with and through the issues and the behaviours that arise. This process needs to be consistent, non-punitive and must not avoid, reject or disregard the underlying issues. Bion (1962) described it as an active process that involves feeling, thinking, organising and acting to enable the distress to be managed appropriately and effectively.

---

and is, in fact, self-destructive and traumatising for both staff and service users and therefore it is an unethical and unacceptable basis for social care structures. I would like to examine and explore these issues, concentrating upon the theoretical underpinnings of relational security and organisational containment, the tensions between managerial and clinical anxieties, the preference for certain clinical models over others and the social and ethical implications involved. The NPM model elevates individual over group advantage and essentially denies the importance of the political, cultural and social context as a major factor in the success or failure of health and social care systems. The theoretical underpinnings of this position need to be challenged.

The individual and the group

The notion of an individual person with a core sense of self as some sort of fixed, predominantly internalised container, separated from others subjectively, is a deeply embedded conception. It is an understandable but limited perception.

Group analytic theory holds that:

> The individual is an artificial, though plausible, abstraction; each person is basically and centrally determined by the world in which he or she lives: by the group: by the community of which he or she forms a part. Inside and outside, individual and society, body and mind, fantasy and reality, cannot be opposed. All separation is artificial isolation. The individual is a part of a

social network, 'a little nodal point as it were', and can only artificially be considered in isolation, like a fish out of water.

(Pines, Hearst & Behr, 1982, p. 139)

S. H. Foulkes (1964), the founder of Group Analysis, saw the need to articulate a new theory of mind to accommodate the social and relational view of human beings and emphasise our essential interconnectedness. This is not to say that the social or group to which one belongs takes precedence or is elevated above the individual. In essence the focus is upon our interdependency. The individual, through active participation in the group, always remains the central focus and the optimal degree of liberation and integration of the individual is paramount in that we all possess a sense of unique subjectivity, psychological insight and agency. The aim is to consider the relationship between the individual and the social group as intrinsically and actively linked together dialogically in meaningful interaction. This is an open-ended, emergent process which requires a safe-enough containing context to thrive, integrating and promoting healthy biological and social processes. Winnicott's facilitating and maturational environment (1965), Bion's container/contained (1962) and Vygotsky's zone of proximal development (1978) provide a foundation for this understanding. If, as Winnicott suggests, there is no essential separation in early life between the mother and infant but only a reciprocal dyadic relationship, then this is also the case with the individual and the group, the person and their community. Someone presenting with a mental health problem should not be seen as only bringing a separate individual problem. Their problem represents only one aspect of an intricate and complex social/group phenomenon. Individual disturbances should be located in all the aspects of a person's life and in their network of interpersonal relationships. We cannot conceptualise or consider individuals as if they were in isolation from the formative, social and cultural context in which they live and work.

This model, as Kerr states (2009): 'needs to incorporate a semiotically-informed, "socio-psycho developmental" dimension in order adequately to account for individual and collective, human health and well-being, or, distress and dysfunction.'

Similarly, E. O. Wilson, the founder of socio-biology, in his recent book *The Meaning of Human Existence,* points us towards the group/psycho-biological understanding of evolutionary development rather than one based on individual fitness. Wilson argues that while selfish activity within a group provides competitive advantage it is ultimately destructive to group welfare as a whole: 'Within groups selfish individuals beat altruistic individuals, but groups of altruists beat groups of selfish individuals or, risking oversimplification, individual selection promoted sin, while group selection promoted virtue' (Wilson, 2014, p. 33).

The NPM model

The neo-liberal/managed care model (NPM) is based upon a cultural paradigm formed from a view promoting the primacy of the individual over social needs. The cultural paradigm lying behind this view is rooted in the belief that unfettered free enterprise, elevating self-interest over social needs will optimally organise every facet of society, including economic and social life. This is a belief system founded upon empirical scientific principles that conclude that the nature of reality can be understood by behavioural and materialistic theories discoverable by evidence-based research, such as randomised control trials. Of course, evidence-based approaches are not bad per se, it is rather how the 'evidence' is construed and how alternative approaches or models are dismissively excluded which is problematic. The validity of the 'evidence based' research culture is examined and challenged elsewhere in this book and, in support, I would argue that this particular approach is based upon a series of dogmas which fuel a fantasy of discovering a 'perfect', all-encompassing understanding of how we function together, dangerously over-objectifying and reducing, rather than valuing, what is human.

There is a considerable body of evidence supporting the view of human beings and their well-being and effectiveness as being developmentally socially formed and located (Ormay, 2012; Gantt & Badenoch, 2013; Brown & Zinkin, 1994; Pines, 2002: Stern, 2000; Trevarthen & Aitken, 2001; Kerr, 2009), although this is largely disregarded by proponents of individualist, neo-liberal ideologies. As a basis for social care systems, NPM fosters a cultural context where health and well-being becomes commodified and the human relational elements, which are intrinsic to care, become devalued. Tasks are organised with other aims in mind and this can create a climate which distances clinicians from each other and from personal contact with their patients. We get a health care ethos which, at its worst, turns patients into demanding and potentially litigious consumers, and clinicians into alienated production line workers. In its attempt to reduce anxiety and risk, it actually does the opposite and creates conditions which perversely cause trauma, resentment and a reactive defensiveness which inhibit the very thing it purports to deliver (Hoggett, 2010; Long, 2009). Through inadequate or neglectful inattention (neo-liberal economic theory) or reactive, abrupt and controlling attention (bureaucratic, top-down management protocols) the NPM business model creates unhealthy working relations and leaves staff deeply insecure and struggling to survive and thrive. Like the neglectful, indifferent parent who overreacts to their unruly, uncontained children, managers, infected by neo-liberal principles, will invariably resort to over-controlling, punitive measures to ensure compliance. Interestingly, the first country to implement neo-liberal economic policy in the 1970s was Chile, which was run by a military dictatorship following the US-led overthrow of a democratically elected socialist government.

The culture of the NHS has been drastically altered over the past two decades as this model has been implemented. For instance, to serve this structural change, there has been an explosion in middle managerial jobs largely at the expense of clinical ones and, as a consequence, this has seen a large increase in the pursuit of 'targets' and bureaucratic imperatives. As the drive for competitive 'success' trundles on, promoted by centralised directives designed to increase efficiency and throughput, pressures upon the clinical staff increase to fulfil what seem like incomprehensible and clinically irrelevant bureaucratic tasks, which, notwithstanding the necessity for properly evaluated practice (Roth & Fonagy, 2005), are extraneous, unnecessary and stultifying. A disparity develops between the aims of the managers and administrators and those of clinicians. This is experienced as an imposition from above with little apparent concern for what is actually required to address the pressures of managing the clinical work. Staff stress is increased and levels of anxiety are raised. For instance, our anxiety increases if we are asked or required to do something we are unable to do because the conditions and the context of the working environment conspire to thwart us in the task. This can lead to situations where financial cuts are implemented in the name of efficiency, and staff are still expected to maintain the same work levels with fewer resources available. If overstretched and overworked staff are asked to achieve unrealistic targets or are compelled to do clinically irrelevant paperwork, if staff are put into situations which leave them feeling impotent and traumatised in the face of patient needs by reducing the type or length of treatments against their professional judgement, then, of course, anxiety will increase. If we sanction a health care system based on a business model where profit is the motive that determines the efficiency or is the rationale for decisions on resources, we get one where the pressures to reduce financial costs triumphs over ethical, professional and clinical judgement. If we sanction a health care system where financial incentives are the priority, we get a system which is likely to become less concerned about staff and patient needs and more likely to cut corners to maximise profit. We only need to look at what is happening with homecare for the elderly and disabled where the worst aspects of privatised healthcare are allowed to place profit over patients. In late 2014 the *Key to Care* report presented an account of the working life of a typical homecare worker. It showed that they are overworked and underpaid, have very little time to maintain a meaningful relationship with care users and some care users were seen by 50 different people in one year. The report stated:

> As publicly funded care continues to be squeezed the danger is that good providers are driven out, and those providers who make a profit by exploiting workers thrive. The price of poor care is paid for by the most vulnerable in our community, and by the care workers they rely who get a raw deal. We must make care work a career of esteem, where a living wage is paid, staff are trained and recognised as key workers who contribute a huge amount to society. This will inevitably come at a price, but the cost of doing nothing will be even greater.

The NHS, as enshrined in the Beveridge report (1942) was created as a model for social care and welfare systems. It has traditionally and symbolically been seen as a good enough, surrogate mother caring for the nation's health from 'the cradle to the grave'. In one of the discussions at the Creating a Healthier NHS meeting it was suggested that, at the present time, it looks as if she is now a desperate, failing mother struggling, with limited resources, to look after the family, while the father (state) is detaching himself from her, more concerned about possible alimony payments when the divorce comes through while spending most of his time dallying with his mistress (private healthcare) (Wilke & Blackwell, 2014). Attention to this is becoming increasingly more important as the new commissioning groups are now actively tendering out services to private healthcare companies. This process is likely to be further reinforced and perpetuated by the impending Transatlantic Trade Investment Partnership discussions between the European Union and the United States.

Organisational anxiety

Much of the anxiety we experience is appropriate. Personal and social well-being or distress cannot be located outside of the social and cultural context in which we live and, at the present time, we live in an anxious age, the age of 'austerity', the age of 'affluenza' (James, 2007), relentlessly urged on by the massive informational output of the media and advertising. Disingenuously, 'austerity' measures are justified as a necessary response to excessive public spending rather than to the failures of the free market boom and bust, the neo-liberal agenda. The anxiety and distress of these are borne, not by those with protected, vested interests, but by the general population and public services. Additionally, we are all subject to our own personal and social dramas and tragedies which are anxiety provoking and, as James contends, much of the emotional distress we currently experience is best understood as a reasonable and rational response to the sickness and dysfunction generated by the social conditions in which we live. These are not based upon irrational fears, and it would be irrational not to be anxious at these times. However, as we must continue to live as best we can, it is important that we do not let ourselves be overwhelmed by anxiety, leading to panic or collapse. As this is a vital, individual self-regulating strategy for survival, so too should it be in the context of our professional, working lives. This is particularly important if we work in the caring professions, where we need to be able to manage and contain the anxiety of our patients as well as our own. This can be an onerous task. We cannot ask the staff to hold and contain the anxieties of those in their care if they themselves do not feel held and contained, encouraged and supported by the organisations for whom they work.

The genesis of organisational anxiety, like individual anxiety, is based upon the fear of things going out of control, of fragmentation and collapse and, all too prevalently in the current climate, of disciplinary action, referral to registering bodies, other punishments and sanctions and fear of loss of employment. Organisational change is by its very nature anxiety provoking. As mistakes and problems occur and innovations and new developments arise, this will generate occupational and personal anxiety. As Hopper and colleagues (2012), show, this will invariably manifest itself as 'traumatic', particularly if the underlying structures, in their conception and subsequent operational development, are intrinsically dysfunctional and neglectful in terms of their impact upon human relational dynamics. The NPM model, in my view, exemplifies this as it strives to place profit above people and imposes bureaucratic protocols and procedures above clinical need and efficacy.

In social care systems organisational anxiety manifests itself in the fear of failed treatment outcomes, services not achieving stated aims, inadequate resources compared with demands, frequent complaints and serious incidents. All of this affects staff morale. Competent managers should know that without winning hearts and minds and the commitment of employees, an organisation will do badly in these circumstances. When high levels of anxiety are experienced, staff distress can lead to situations which are potentially self-destructive. The high profile case of the nurse who inadvertently transferred a telephone call enquiring about a member of the Royal family to presenters on an Australian radio programme and, tragically, chose to take her own life rather than face the consequences, is an example of this unbearable personal distress.

The setting

In social care systems the context is all important. In my experience, if you get the context right then you optimise the treatment outcome and therapeutic potential. This applies, not only in mental health settings but is equally appropriate to other contexts in the NHS with obvious variations depending upon local and clinical circumstances. The safety of the consulting room, the ward, the community team or GP practice, is paramount. It must be safe enough for the work to be carried out effectively. A supportive setting must be created that is safe enough for our patients to begin to trust us and take risks as the treatment or therapeutic process and attachment to clinicians and services goes through the different phases of illness to wellness. Also, we must have these conditions in place if we are to manage the inevitable distress when things do not go well.

The setting has to feel physically as well as emotionally safe. For instance, at the most basic level, services and spaces in which social/healthcare takes place must be clean, comfortable and familiar and, most importantly, there should be a continuity of care received from a relationship with familiar and known staff. In most GP practices or out-patient clinics the only regularly known person will be the receptionist. Most of us would like to be seen by the same GP or consultant with whom we can establish a personal relationship. This feels safer than meeting someone new each time we have an appointment. This, unfortunately, tends to be the common experience many of us currently face as we access health and social care. When we are anxious and concerned about our physical or mental health we are vulnerable and frightened. At these times we need to feel held and contained (looked after) to enable us to stay with the difficult process we are going through. Good human relationships based on consistency and continuity, underpinned and informed by what John Ballatt and Penelope Campling call 'Intelligent Kindness' (2012) is what is required at these times, not fragmented, transitory contact with different people or services. Ballatt and Campling's compelling book comprehensively outlines in more depth the views I am arguing for and I would urge anyone working in or concerned about how we manage social care to read it.

Of primary concern is the welfare of the staff undertaking the work. Most people who choose to go into social care work are motivated to help others and, therefore themselves, as they contribute to the greater welfare of the community to which they belong. Many are also to some extent 'wounded healers' bearing their own difficult, but motivating, formative experiences. This may helpfully render such professionals particularly attuned and committed to patients but also can make them liable to suffer badly if subjected to such experiences again at the hands of an adversarial and toxic management system. If the basic underpinnings of the structure, the foundation upon which it stands or falls – the staff – are not seen as primary, if their welfare is not given priority, then this raises questions about the quality of the work undertaken and highlights the all too apparent dangers evident in the high levels of staff sickness, absence, burnout and distress which currently plague many services.

Organisational containment and relational security

Organisational containment is a rather mysterious notion, not easily conveyed. It involves a sense of calmness, reassurance and familiarity that permeates the space within which work is undertaken, including the building in which work takes place and the wider environment, both psychologically and physically (Simpson, 1995). In my experience, this can defuse potentially damaging situations much more effectively than putting security locks on doors or having panic buttons in the rooms. It is essential that the impulse to overreact defensively or protectively is not given its head. For instance, constant organisational change, which, in itself, provokes massive anxieties each time it is implemented, is a good example of this and as anyone who works in the NHS knows, this is often the management's response to solving service problems. Some time ago Isobel Menzies Lyth (1959) showed the fallacy of this, but generally little attention has been paid to such issues.

If ontological security (Laing, 1965) (that is, a solid, core sense of self, which is separate and autonomous yet intrinsically and relationally linked to others, acknowledging the difference and managing the ever-present tension of being overwhelmed or ostracised by the group) is the goal of the individual, then relational security, a term recently promoted by the Department of Health, initially directed towards mental health wards in forensic settings, should be the goal for social care systems. The Department of Health booklet *See, Think and Act* (2010) defines it as follows: Relational security is the knowledge and understanding staff have of a patient and of the environment; and the translation of that information into appropriate response and care.

This is a laudable aim, without question, but its implementation can often be skewed by a defensive overreaction from the management, who misinterpret the need to respond and start top down, managed procedures aimed at reducing the risk to the wider organisational status rather than attending to the needs and concerns of the frontline staff who are expected to establish and maintain such relational security.

When we consider a set of principles which should be in place in any organisation involved in all social care systems it is important that these are informed by a bio-psycho-social understanding (Engel, 1977). Choosing between either medical or psychological approaches is a false choice. Physical distress always has a psychological meaning and context. Any response to distress (including medical) conveys a psychological attitude and impact. Psychological understanding is therefore a prerequisite for coherent, sensible planning. This applies to acute hospitals, social service departments and all the other agencies, voluntary or otherwise, whose remit is to care for people, not just provide mental health services. For instance, it is professionally unacceptable that staff, working in community mental health teams, have caseloads that are so large that they cannot hold the service users in mind. Similarly, it is unacceptable, when services are reorganised, to inform staff only two weeks before changes take place that they must end their relationship with their patients, which may have been established over a long period. This is no way to handle important or personally significant endings. The intrinsic value of human relational contact and the emotional significance of this is ignored and denied. This is also the case in acute hospital settings where staff are not adequately trained, supervised and supported in dealing with the emotional turmoil experienced with patients who are ill or dying. If we accept this, if we support this, it is unethical if we do not put these principles into place, or even fight to put them into place, in mental health and social and medical settings.

Where understanding is absent or service practices are governed by a misconceived view, this can lead to personal and organisational assumptions that staff should somehow manage the tensions and anxieties generated as if it did not affect them adversely at times. Sharing and containing pain and suffering is distressing. If we fail to do this in a professionally appropriate way, defensive measures emerge to safeguard self-esteem and perverse patterns can develop as containing mechanisms. The emergence of a perverse organisational solution, as Rosemary Rizq argues, can result in a culture:

> where these anxieties are concealed and disavowed beneath a fetishised 'target culture' which offers an idealised picture of the work of a mental health service whilst simultaneously undermining and subverting the very care that it is mandated by government to provide.
>
> *(Rizq, 2014, p. 255)*

Rizq also proposes that the UK government's current response to this situation is one:

> in which it is not only implementing a large-scale mental health policy based on improving financial productivity in a time of unprecedented global austerity, (thereby 'turning a blind eye' to contemporary global socio-economic realities) but one in which the dependency and psychological suffering of patients, as well as the anxieties and limitations of those tasked

with caring for them are simultaneously disavowed and concealed beneath overwhelming bureaucratic and governance systems.

(Rizq, 2014, p. 262)

In social care services, the basic issue is the tension between capacity and demand, especially in times of reduced resources. This can lead to day-to-day professional and ethical dilemmas about how to exercise a realistic and proper duty of care. The inevitable levels of anxiety this generates throughout an organisation creates a volatile situation. When capacity is reduced, demand increases as waiting lists get longer, services become stretched, staff can feel pressurised, resentful and embittered and the possibility of incidents and abusive responses increase. In the face of inappropriate professionalism due to distress and suffering or lack of understanding about underlying societal dysfunction and the inability to enable and maintain appropriate commitment and humanity by overstretched and disillusioned staff, creates potentially dangerous situations. The abuses which took place in Mid Staffordshire and Winterbourne View are examples of the consequences when things get out of control in this way. In this situation, within the current NPM paradigm and its culture of misguided and misinformed 'managerialism' (Jarman, 2012) an organisation can look for solutions by concentrating on the wrong areas. Even though the Francis report (2013) advocated the need for better staff support, the response of many organisations was to increase the top down surveillance. Rather than look at underpinning the infrastructure for the staff – their safety and support as the most important factors – the organisation attempts to manage the heightened anxiety levels by over-controlling the policy and procedural structure. As organisations grapple with these issues they can become 'traumatised' themselves and 'traumatising' towards their staff, at all levels in the structure. Chris Scanlon and John Adlam, in a seminar paper, Scanlon and Adlam (2012) show how staff working in traumatised organisations there is a powerful oscillation between the distress and demandingness of clients below, and what is experienced as the restrictions and controls from management above.

When this occurs, an organisation can disregard the most valuable element in the clinical process and lose sight of the understanding that working with mental or physical distress is best addressed through good staff support initiatives rather than through the implementation of procedural mechanisms. Unless staff welfare and support is emphasised and established as a primary concern, the importance of all aspects of the working context will remain sadly unacknowledged and undervalued and the management of the anxiety generated in the working setting will not be fully understood or addressed. If relational security in the workplace is to mean anything it must be focused on staff support and welfare. In situations when management loses this focus and is reactive rather than reflective, this can mean a loss of the human dimension and an inappropriate over-reliance on protocols and procedures, reinforced by an unhelpful and threatening culture of 'discipline' and punishment. In a social care service setting this is highlighted in the tensions between the management and clinical anxiety.

Management and clinical anxiety

I am indebted to the work of R. D. Hinshelwood, who highlighted the distinction between managerial and clinical anxiety. Acknowledging this difference draws attention to the likelihood of a basic and structural misunderstanding about how to contain and manage anxiety depending upon the position from which it is viewed.

As Hinshelwood points out; the consequence is that managerial anxiety is likely to leak into the clinical situation, with the potential for overload, and a decline in clinical performance rather than an improvement (Hinshelwood, 1994, p. 290).

While individual clinicians struggle with the personal and emotional effects of change, in terms of relational dynamics and the consequences for themselves and those in their care, managers have priorities determined by wider organisational policy directed from above. They too are located in their own particular world of meaning and significance. They are concerned about their personal and professional need to be approved and valued by peers and their own management. While the overarching organisational aim may be to create and maintain a viable, efficient and effective health care system, their priorities, because of operational pressures, will not always coincide with those of clinicians on the frontline. This disparity is particularly damaging in a management culture informed and motivated by neo-liberal economic theory. In these circumstances, management anxiety will invariably focus on resource allocation, budget setting, the application of systems or structures for compliance in terms of target setting, data collection, increased activity or efficiencies and clinical governance procedures. And, although many managers are well meaning and set out with best of intentions, such a culture unfortunately also encourages and promotes individuals with underlying authoritarian personality structures who can all too easily turn into bullies who may enact their own psychological agendas of envy, retribution and vengefulness towards clinicians and other professionals. When anxiety permeates an overburdened, overstretched service, the disparity between managerial and clinical anxiety becomes all too apparent. The disconnect between the two positions can result in staff feeling devalued as if their clinical concerns are of secondary importance while managers justify their position by highlighting the need for efficiencies through cost improvement plans. In these circumstances, management proposals can seem censorious, undermining or punitive.

The concentration upon prohibitive and time consuming processes, which reduce face-to-face clinical time and increase paranoid anxieties around blame and censure, closes down the possibility of creative, professional solutions between clinicians and supervisees and clinicians and their patients. As clinical staff struggle with the day-to-day anxieties of managing and containing patient distress and disturbance they also end up resentful and disaffected, feeling uncontained or unsupported themselves by the wider organisational structure. Patients too become the victims of this approach as treatment models are also devalued because they are considered uneconomical or wasteful. Shorter models are valued above longer term ones irrespective of the consequences for those with complex and difficult presentations.

Layard's (2006) vision to improve access to psychological treatments is a commendable aim but it has been hijacked by those advocating one particular clinical model. The predominance of cognitive behavioural therapy as the panacea for mental distress sustains the fantasy that society's ills can be contained within one limited model and views them as technical problems or medical illnesses, as if they were individual problems divorced or separate from the social culture and context within which they occur (Rizq, 2014).

Of course, it is important that social care services have clinical and other governance protocols in place. However, these processes should always be directed and informed from the bottom up, focusing primarily on staff and patient relational dynamics, not from top down attempts to improve production quotas or reactive strategies which increase mistrust. Managerial directives requiring clinicians to write up and record every supervision session rather than trust that the relational process within a 'good enough' supervision setting is trustworthy and robust, is an example of this. Emphasis is placed upon superficial, rigid, procedural formats which, although their aim is supposedly transparency and openness, make those involved feel that they are not to be trusted unless a record is kept of everything that transpires. Not only does this involve extra paperwork and less time spent working clinically but it also constrains rather than frees up exploration and discovery.

If an NHS Trust's status and financial resources are dependent upon achieving government-led targets, the organisation becomes, and this has been borne out in my own experience, preoccupied with the avoidance of wider organisational censure and blame and it will more often than not pass these anxieties down on to individual clinical services. For instance, the anxiety generated by risky, difficult patients, their management and the inevitable incidents which can follow, are often interpreted within the wider organisational setting as a vehicle to highlight or single out particular services or ways of working as examples of inadequate or inferior practice. This action enhances splits and fragmentation rather than integration and cohesiveness. Group analytic theory points out how groups behave in times of high anxiety by attempting to locate anxiety provoking difficulties onto a particular location or individual in the hope that by locating the problem there a resolution can be found either by removing them or sanctioning them. This is the classic scapegoat motif and, of course, it misses the basic point that the difficulty is a wider, group relational problem and must be addressed by the organisation as a whole. If it is placed in one location, generally all that happens is there is some temporary relief, but the basic issue is not addressed or acknowledged. As a result, as time passes, the problem will arise again and this pattern will repeat itself. The difficulty here is in not fully recognising or acknowledging that under-resourced and over-stretched services are trying to manage the inherent risk involved in the containment of difficult or highly distressed patients as if isolated or separated out from the wider organisational dynamic. In essence, it should be seen as a whole system problem, not just one for particular services, although there may be issues that a particular service could improve in any given circumstance. Obholzer and Roberts make this point, when they say:

Systems which encourage open discussion of work-related feelings and problems, in a climate which regards 'problems' as a normal aspect of the work rather than as evidence of personal or group pathology, encourage individual and organisational learning, and can thus foster growth and development.

(Obholzer & Roberts, 1994, p. 208)

Staff support and the containment of anxiety

Anxiety is always with us. It is a part of our human condition. It cannot be eradicated to create an anxiety free state. However, at best, we can create conditions in which we can minimise anxiety and help ourselves manage and deal with it as it emerges in our lives. In our desire to hold ourselves together at these times when anxiety levels are high, we are likely to employ the most primitive attempt to manage overwhelming anxiety by defensive measures. Early, ongoing good enough experiences of containment, active support, encouragement, appreciation, recognition, joint participation in common worthwhile endeavours enable us to develop the ability to manage experiences and emotion. When these are inadequate or significantly interrupted, cognitive and emotional development are adversely affected. This is no less so in the workplace. Therefore, a co-regulating, healthy, socially informed interaction between those caring for and those cared for is essential for safety and security.

The essential requirements of a model applicable to all social care systems must take as its primary aim the welfare and support of the staff who undertake the work. Therefore they should be valued for the contribution they make by being adequately resourced personally and professionally. Their pay and conditions should reflect this and they should be provided with a safe enough context at work. This means they should have adequate and appropriate training and, more importantly, they should be in regular clinical supervision, preferably in groups, as well as having line management supervision. This should apply to managers too as this would help them to better understand the clinical dynamics involved. Similarly, all staff (including managers, directors and chief executives) should have an externally facilitated, regular reflective practice space available to them which provides the opportunity to explore together the affects working in social care has upon them. The merits of reflective practice are well documented (Simpson, 2010; Carson & Dennison, 2008; Thorndycraft & Mc Cabe, 2008; Hesse, 2001; Bramley, 1990; Rifkind, 1995) and, in my view, this is an essential precondition for healthy survival in social care systems.

Concluding remarks

While recognising and acknowledging that financial priorities are important and that they will necessarily be limited by resource and budget limitations, I would argue that if we are once again to aspire to the founding principles of a national health service, this should not be directed by an individualistically oriented, neo-liberal business model but should be underpinned by a more socially integrated and coherent understanding of the essential nature of human relationship and their interdependence. If we are to put a comprehensive structure in place for social care we should have a progressive taxation framework established which adequately funds the NHS and other social care services. A statutory, national service for the public, free at the point of delivery and based upon need rather than the ability to pay should be the aim. Limited resources and the establishing and developing of appropriate support structures for staff and patients are not mutually exclusive. In the long run, if a social care system properly informed by an understanding of clinical and ethical priorities, not the desire for profit or efficiency targets, is established, this will not only pay for itself in financial terms but, over time, will help create a robust, fair and equitable work setting which optimises patient wellbeing and health. I have no desire to over-idealise the function of the welfare state or suggest that the model I argue for will provide 'perfect' care. On the contrary, I would rather see it as an emergent 'work in progress' which acknowledges and recognises the complex struggle involved in establishing a social care system based upon equity and fairness and not upon profits or for the benefit of a privileged minority. It is always going to be difficult to manage anxiety in the NHS and associated health and social care systems, vulnerable as they are to the ideological battles between the different political parties. Perhaps, like the Bank of England, health and social care should be taken out of the hands of politicians and given a different, favoured, protected status with social and egalitarian aims in place and with adequate and appropriate financial resources allocated to ensure stability and security. This would make health and social care systems safer for all concerned and insulate them from most of the disturbing changes they have been subjected to in the recent past.

References

Ballatt, J. & Campling, P. (2011). *Intelligent kindness: Reforming the culture of healthcare.* London: RCPsych.

Beveridge Report (1942). London: H.M.S.O.

Bion, W. R. (1970). *Attention and interpretation.* London: Tavistock.

Bramley, W. (1990). Staff sensitivity groups: A conductor's field of experiences. *Group Analysis, 23*(3), 301–16.

Brown, D. & Zinkin, L. (1994). *The psyche and the social world: Developments in group analytic theory.* London: Routledge.

Burstow Commission (2014). *Key to care: Report to the Burstow commission on the future of the homecare workforce.* Local Government Information Unit.

Carson, J. & Dennison, P. (2008). The role of groupwork in tackling organisational burnout: Two contrasting perspectives. *Groupwork, 18*(2), 18–25.

Department of Health (DoH) (2007). *Commissioning for a brighter future: Improving access to psychological therapies. Positive practice guide.* London: Department of Health.

Department of Health Booklet. (2010). *See, think and act: Your guide to relational security.* London: Department of Health.

Dobson, A. (2007). *Green Political Thought.* London: Routledge.

Engel, G. L. (1977). The need for a new medical model: A challenge for biomedicine. *Science, 196,* 129–36.

Foulkes, S. H. (1964). *Therapeutic group analysis.* London: George Allen & Unwin.

Francis, R. (2013). *The Mid Staffordshire NHS foundation trust public inquiry.* London: The Stationery Office.

Gantt, S. P. & Badenoch, B. (eds) (2013). *The interpersonal neurobiology of group psychotherapy and group process.* London, Karnac.

Griffiths, R. (1983). Report on the NHS. Socialist Health Association Website. Available at: www.sochealth.co.uk/national-health-service/griffiths-report-october-1983, accessed 01 October 2015.

Hesse, N. (2001). The function and value of staff groups on a psychiatric ward. *Psychoanalytic Psychotherapy, 15,* 121–30.

Hinshelwood, R. D. (1994). The relevance of psychotherapy. *Psychoanalytic Psychotherapy, 8*(3), 290.

Hoggett, P. (2010). Government and the perverse social defence. *British Journal of Psychotherapy, 26,* 202–12.

Hood, C. (1991). A public management for all seasons. *Public Administration, 69,* 3–19.

Hopper, E. (ed.) (2012). *Trauma and organisations.* London: Karnac Books.

James, O. (2007). *Affluenza.* London: Vermillion.

Jarman, B. (2012). When managers rule. *British Medical Journal, 345,* e8239.

Kerr, I. (2009). Addressing the socially-constituted self through a common language for mental health and social service: A cognitive-analytic perspective. In J. Forbes & C. Watson (eds), *Confluences of identity, knowledge and practice: building interprofessional social capital. ESCR Seminar Proceedings (4), Research Paper, 20,* (pp. 21–38). Aberdeen, UK: University of Aberdeen.

Krugman, P. (2012). *End this depression now.* New York: W.W. Norton.

Laing, R. (1965). *The divided self.* London: Pelican.

Layard, R. (2006). The depression report: A new deal for depression and anxiety disorders. London: LSE.

Lister, J. (2013). *The neoliberal epidemic striking healthcare.* Available at: www.opendemocracy.net/ournhs, accessed 7 June 2013.

Long, S. (2009). Greed. *Psychodynamic Practice, 15,* 245–59.

Menzies Lyth, I. (1960). A case-study in the functioning of social systems as a defence against anxiety: A report on the study of the nursing services of a general hospital. *Human Relations, 13,* 95–121.

Obholzer, A. & Roberts, V. Z. (1994). *The unconscious at work: Individual and organisational stress in the human services.* London: Routledge.

Ormay, A. P. (2012). *The social nature of persons: One person is no person.* London: Karnac.

Piketty, T. (2014). *Capital in the twenty-first century.* Cambridge, MA: Harvard University Press.

Pines, M. (2002). The coherency of group analysis. *Group Analysis, 35*(I), 13–26. London: Sage.

Pines, M., Hearst, L. & Behr, H. L. (1982). Group analysis (group analytic psychotherapy). In G. M. Gazda (ed.), *Basic approaches to group psychotherapy and group counselling* (pp. 132–78). Springfield, IL: Thomas.

Reid, J. (1972). *Speech at Glasgow University in 1972.* University of Glasgow, UK. Reprinted in the *Independent,* 13 August 2010.

Rifkind, G. (1995). Containing the containers: The staff consultation group. *Group Analysis, 28,* 209–22.

Rizq, R. (2014). Perverting the course of therapy: The fetishisation of governance in public sector mental health services. *Psychoanalytic Psychotherapy, 28*(3), 249–67.

Roth, T. & Fonagy, P. (2005). *What works for whom: A critical review of psychotherapy research* (2nd edn). New York & London: Guilford Press.

Scanlon, C. & Adlam, J. (2012). On the (dis)stressing effects of working in (dis)stressed homelessness organisations. *Journal of Housing Care, Care and Support* (Special Edition on Psychologically Informed Environments), *15*(2): 74–82.

Simpson, I. (1995). Group therapy within the NHS: We all know about 'good enough' but is it 'safe enough? *Group Analysis, 28*, 223–35.

Simpson, I. (2010). Containing the uncontainable: A role for staff support groups. In J. Radcliffe, K. Hajek, J. Carson & O. Manor (eds), *Psychological groupwork with acute psychiatric inpatients* (pp. 87–105). London: Whiting & Birch.

Stern, D. (2000). *The interpersonal world of the infant: A view from psychoanalysis and developmental psychology* (2nd edn). New York, NY: Basic Books.

Stieglitz, J. (2012). *The price of inequality*. New York: W.W. Norton.

Thorndycraft, B. & Mc Cabe, J. (2008). The challenge of working with staff groups in the caring professions: The importance of the 'Team Development and Reflective Practice Group.' *British Journal of Psychotherapy, 24*(2), 167–83.

Trevarthen, C. & Aitken, K. J. (2001). Infant intersubjectivity: Research, theory and clinical applications. *Journal of Child Psychology & Psychiatry, 42*, 3–48.

Wilke, G. & Blackwell, D. (November 2014). Discussion at Creating a Healthier NHS meeting.

Wilkinson, R. & Pickett, K. (2009). *The spirit level: Why more equal societies almost always do better*. London: Allen Lane.

Wilson, O. E. (2014). *The meaning of human existence*. New York: Liveright.

Winnicott, D. W. (1976). *The maturational processes and the facilitating environment*. London: Hogarth Press and Institute of Psycho-Analysis.

Vygotsky, L. (1978). *Mind in society: The development of higher psychological processes*. Cambridge, MA: Harvard University Press.

6

STATES OF ABJECTION IN MANAGED CARE[1]

Rosemary Rizq

Introduction

In a recent meeting, a group of colleagues and I were discussing a young woman who had been referred to our National Health Service (NHS) primary care mental health service. This young woman was experiencing an episode of quite severe depression and had gone to her doctor seeking psychotherapeutic help. In the letter from the doctor, we learned that she had experienced a number of problems since early childhood: she had initially been raised in foster care; abused by a neighbour, she had left home at only 17, and subsequently engaged in a series of emotionally and sexually abusive relationships with men. The father of her baby had recently been jailed for drug-related crime, and now, at 24, she was raising her two-year-old by herself. She was currently unemployed, struggling to manage on government benefits and appeared to have no family and few support networks available. The GP was clearly very concerned about her and was putting the service under considerable pressure to treat her as a matter of priority.

During the discussion, a disagreement between various members of the group turned into a full-scale debate about the nature of the service, what it should be offering the community and the criteria for accepting patients into the service. While one or two clinicians, including myself, felt that it was possible to offer this young woman some focused, brief work to address the current problem, the majority, including the clinical lead, felt that this patient's history meant that this was unlikely to be helpful. A number of anxieties were raised about the value of the brief psychotherapeutic work that would be available: Suppose the patient regressed? How could the service manage and contain the probable risk issues? If ongoing support was needed pending any necessary referral to the community mental health team, how would this be reflected in targets and staff activity data, already under scrutiny by senior management? In the course of this lengthy debate, one of my colleagues, by now no doubt tired and exasperated, asked whether we thought the service was simply there to deal with 'shit life syndrome'. This rather vivid rhetorical question resulted, unsurprisingly, in some further heated discussion, which was eventually cut short by the clinical lead who agreed that, despite pressure from the doctor to accept this patient, the service could indeed not afford to take on everyone who suffered from 'shit life syndrome', and took the decision to reject the referral.

I have since become very curious about this expression 'shit life syndrome', not the least because of the implicit consensus by everyone in the meeting, including myself, as to what it meant. The phrase seemed to denote a level of long-standing poverty, family breakdown, lack of stability, unemployment and potential risk factors common to many of the predominantly young, working class patients referred to the service. There was no doubt that, quite apart from important debates about the inclusion and exclusion criteria for the service, these issues aroused a number of un-spoken anxieties in all of us present at the meeting. But the particular choice of words used by my colleague I think tells us something about the unconscious nature of these anxieties. For shit, of course, is something that we generally prefer not to think about; something we continually reject, get rid of or hide. At the same time, it is something that we cannot completely repudiate; it is part of us, something we need, something that is ineluctably part of our status as human beings, as subjects. Those suffering from 'shit-life syndrome', then, would seem to be those individuals whose problems are deemed to be so terrible, so untouchable, that they quite literally cannot be thought about, cannot be handled by the service. At the same time, the organiza-tion is obliged to do so; it is confronted by continual pressure from the public and from referrers to provide psychological care and treatment for these same individuals who arouse such intense anxiety and from whom its staff wish to distance themselves.

In bringing a psychoanalytic sensibility to the study of organizations, Gabriel and Carr (2002) suggest that it 'opens valuable windows into the world of organiza-tions and management, offering insights that are startlingly original, have extensive explanatory powers and can find ample practical implementations' (p. 348). While much psychoanalytic thinking about organizational dynamics traditionally draws on the object relations theories of Klein (1946) and Bion (1962), in this chapter I want to consider Kristeva's (1982) notion of the abject as a possible alternative lens through which to think about anxiety within mental health services. Kristeva suggests that anxiety indexes the perpetual attempt by the subject to expel some-thing of the self that is deemed to be repulsive or untouchable, a dynamic that I will suggest has remained significant throughout society's long history of care for the mentally ill.

The arguments in this chapter are located in the context of contemporary UK public mental health services, which have been identified by Thomas and Davies (2005), along with all public sector organizations, as 'sites of transformative change' (p. 684) since the 1980s, as a result of new public management (NPM) restructuring of health, education and social services. A particular emphasis in NPM is the intro-duction of new disciplinary technologies (Townley, 1994) aimed at instilling new organizational attitudes sponsoring workers' compliance with government target systems. These targets, and the technologies designed to generate them, actively construct the organizations in which they operate, shaping the behaviour and subjectivities of staff as well as the public perception of problems for which they are considered to be the solution (Power, 1997). In this chapter, I will attempt to link the unconscious dynamics of abjection with the organizational policies, structures and practices of contemporary UK mental health services subject to these technologies, specifically drawing on my work as a psychotherapist and supervisor within an Improving Access to Psychological Therapies (IAPT) service.

Using the above example as a starting point then, I start by offering a brief introduction to Lacanian and Kristevan views of anxiety before exploring the psychoanalytic notion of social defences in organizations. I then draw on work by Foucault (1964) and Shildrick (2002) to consider how individuals deemed to be psychologically distressed are cast as monstrous or 'other' by society. Exploring the way in which NPM's preoccupations with regulation, surveillance and governance within mental health institutions may be characterized as a symbolic attempt to gain mastery over feelings unconsciously deemed to be abject reminders of the body, I offer an organizational case example to illuminate the way in which abjective dynamics are refracted within one particular IAPT service, impacting on both staff and patients.

Abjection: a theoretical outline

There is no doubt that Kristeva's theories, drawing on psychoanalysis, linguistics, literary theory and philosophy, remain dauntingly abstruse to many clinical practitioners and researchers. Her concept of abjection is well-known to writers on intertextuality (Keenoy & Oswick, 2004; Riad, Vaara, & Zhang, 2012), but is more frequently elaborated by feminist writers concerned with culture, gender and sexuality (e.g. Butler, 2004; Fotaki, 2011; Hopfl, 2008; Tietze, 2003). Her thinking derives from a Lacanian framework in which subjectivity is thought to be consti- tuted by the interweaving of the three psychic realms of the Imaginary, the Symbolic and the Real.[2] In Lacan's (1953) 'mirror stage', his template for the Imaginary order, the child's lack of physical coherence and motor co-ordination, gives rise to a primal anxiety that is only allayed by identification with his or her mirror image. Identification thus confers a subjective feeling of wholeness, completeness and self- mastery, an anticipated sense of self-unity and control that the child does not yet possess. This forms the basis of an imaginary ego, a 'misrecognition' upon which an imaginary identity and thus a psychological dependence on the other is created and sustained. The specular re-constitution of the fragmented body at this stage covers over the ego's basic lack or insufficiency which is experienced as profound anxiety in the face of the Real.

Lacan claims that it is this fundamental loss of the (Imaginary) self that the individual attempts throughout life to recover via language and recognition by the (Symbolic) other. Kristeva (1982) however privileges the maternally oriented, pre- symbolic, pre-linguistic order that she insists precedes, underpins and guarantees the subject of the symbolic order. She sees the mother's body as a receptacle, a place of semiotic drives and boundary-less plenitude. In a symbiotic state, akin to Lacan's Imaginary register, the infant experiences himself as one with and fulfilled by a mother guaranteeing wholeness and unity. In order to enter the Lacanian order of the Symbolic, to become a differentiated subject constituted by language and lack, the subject has to discard the unclean, improper or impure aspects of the maternal body while it is still within this symbiotic tie. The rejected parts of the self 'may be such things as faeces and sour milk, but they may also include symbolic representations of the child's relationship with its mother' (Holmes, Perron & O'Byrne, 2006, p. 307). Kristeva (1982) suggests that feelings of anxiety, disgust, repulsion and fear are ways in which each individual subsequently experiences and attempts to distance him or herself from what is felt to be improper or unclean in order to establish and strengthen his or her own subjectivity and retain a self that is *'propre'* or clean. In this struggle, the maternal body is abjected and becomes the site of primal repression while remaining the seat of maternally oriented psychic energy beneath the symbolic order. Abjection is thus clearly linked to the construction of the speaking subject, where the marginalized or unrepresentable aspects of language, such as the rhythm, prosody and tone of text or speech, are seen to underpin and continually threaten to destabilize the paternally oriented symbolic order governing language, syntax and grammar.

Abjection is thus seen by Kristeva as a process through which the individual's sense of self and corporeal boundaries are established and positioned; where subject and object are distinguished and where toxicity and waste are rejected and order installed. It is the measure by which the subject defines what is 'I' and what is 'not I'. In this struggle, whatever is not clearly demarcated in this way is connoted as abject: 'It is not lack of cleanliness or health that causes abjection' writes Kristeva (1982), 'but what disturbs identity, system, order. What does not respect borders, positions, rules. The in-between, the ambiguous, the composite' (p. 4).

Abjection and the social defence model: anxiety in organizations

Discussions about the role of anxiety within organizations have traditionally been dominated by the so-called 'Tavistock model'. This work draws mainly on Kleinian psychoanalytic thinking to articulate how organizations structure themselves and the subjectivities of staff in order to defend against primitive anxieties. Isabel Menzies-Lyth's (1960) seminal study investigating the reasons for increasing numbers of student nurses leaving the profession found nurses experienced enormous emotional difficulties in handling, working with and caring for the sick, injured and dying patients in their care and argued that such work resurrected primitive anxieties. Her study identified a number of working practices such as strict routines, the division of labour and the identification of patients by number rather than by name that she understood as institutionally embedded defences against death anxiety. Paradoxically, these same social defences reduced nurses' emotional investment in their work and satisfaction in their relationships with patients, ultimately leading to a destabilising level of staff turnover at the hospital.

The Kleinian perspective offered by Menzies-Lyth (1959) and more recent theorists such as Obholzer (2003) also draws on Bion (1962) as a basis for assuming the significance of the institution as a container for the projected feelings and anxieties of society (e.g. Hinshelwood, 1994). However, the defensive position of abjection that Kristeva (1982) describes permits a rather different conceptualization of some of the practices identified by Menzies-Lyth: not simply as institutional defences against a yet-to-be contained anxiety, but rather as part of the institution's enduring efforts to impose symbolic order on an anxiety that can never be completely managed, that is perpetually present and must continually be opposed. The hospital's identification of patients by number rather than by name, the emphasis on ritual, protocol and guidelines and the denial of nurses' feelings and so forth may be seen as an ongoing unconscious attempt by the symbolic to overwrite the semiotic, to control and define the body's boundaries and to regulate the marginalized and unrepresentable aspects of experience in order to safeguard institutional system and order.

What, then, is the relevance of abjection in *psychological* care? In order to address this issue, it is important to remember that the care of the mentally ill has a long and dismaying history, in which their abjection within society has been a constant if tacit dynamic. Foucault (1964) points out that in the Middle Ages, it was the leper who occupied a place on the margins of communities, a space that seemed to open up after leprosy as an illness largely disappeared from the western world. Over the next three centuries, the poor, the criminals and the insane would come to take the place of the leper within society, occupying a liminal position where they were permitted to live in cities, yet were confined within institutions that were intended to control public spaces, clean the streets of 'problem people' and act as correctional establishments to address the economic and social problems emerging from within Europe.

Foucault draws attention to the way in which, from the fifteenth century on, the mentally ill individual was constructed as a 'bestial man . . . the monster who is both man and beast', a construction that legitimated his or her exclusion from society. More recently, Shildrick's (2002) notion of 'monstrosity' drawing on the Lacanian 'mirror stage' in infant development suggests that a sense of our own fragmentation and lack is what we encounter when we see any kind of deformity, disability or damage in others. The modernist ideal of the independent autonomous body and mind is threatened by the recognition that a fundamental lack of unity, an inescapable vulnerability, is the basis of our shared humanity. She goes on to argue that the predictable, 'normal' body is preserved and protected only by a process of normalization that ensures the 'monstrous' other is abjected, marginalized and excluded. In line with Freud's (1919) notion of the 'uncanny', Shildrick (2002) also points to the way in which such a process is implicitly suffused with an anxiety sponsored by the threat of return, the reappearance of the abject:

> Monsters haunt us, not because they represent an external threat – and indeed
> some are benign – but because they stir recognition within, a sense of our open-
> ness and vulnerability that western discourse insists on covering over.
>
> *(p. 81)*

Abjection and contemporary mental health services

The above discussion suggests that the mentally ill or psychologically distressed
individual threatens us with the return of the abject, helping us to define our own
normality and subjectivity by comparison with a radical or 'monstrous' other. This
threat is, of course, particularly salient within mental health services where the
professional role of staff in caring for the mentally ill may be at odds with personal
feelings of unease and vulnerability when faced with those who, as Shildrick (2002)
suggests, unconsciously remind them of their own fragmentation and lack.

It is here that I want to draw attention to the complex interplay between
unconscious dynamics, organizational structure and government health policy.
Recent UK government-backed initiatives such as the IAPT programme can be
seen as both cause and consequence of NPM philosophies that result in organizational structures increasingly characterized by managerialism, surveillance and
bureaucracy. I want to suggest that these 'rituals of verification', typical of the 'audit
society' described by Power (1997) and its logic of coercive accountability, is
constitutive of a mental health service's symbolic attempt to regulate and define
the limits and borders of its own culture, defending the organization and its staff
against the return of the abject.

In line with this view, Hopfl (2003) has argued that organizations have
traditionally been constructed as patriarchal and masculine and that such representations reduce the notion of organizations to abstract relationships, rational action
and purposive behaviour. She contrasts this with a view of the maternally oriented
organization that questions and problematizes the ambivalence that is concealed
and regulated by the patriarchal, symbolic order. Tiezte (2003) similarly points out
that notions of loving, caring, protecting and suffering are intimately linked to
notions of motherhood. 'This very essence of motherhood' she writes, 'is problematic in modern organisations, where the emotive is the abject, the pain of labour
denied, the jouissance and horrors of intimacy rejected' (p. 65).

Tiezte's claim is particularly challenging in the context of the broader welfare
system that Cooper and Lousada (2005) argue constitutes 'a socially-sanctioned
system of concern' (p. 21). They question the way in which 'little reference is
made to intensity of feeling as lying at the heart of the work of welfare' (p. 26)
and point to the paradox that 'day by day the welfare project continues to be about
people, as it always has been and must be. Yet a parallel state of mind has been
created and maintained through its adoption of a position that denies, ignores, and
repudiates this experience' (p. 27).

The rise of NPM strategies of accountability and control within welfare services
in general, and in public mental health services in particular, can thus be seen as
part and parcel of the way in which mental illness and feelings of psychological

distress, along with the vulnerability to which they give rise, are abjected within society and within these organizations. Insofar as the abject is violently expelled from the body, so too I suggest that notions of psychological vulnerability may be violently expelled from the social body that is the organization, that expulsion effectively establishing such feelings as alien, as 'Other'. The ordered, regulated rationality of the Symbolic order expressed by the institution's attempt at regulation, surveillance and governance can be characterized as an attempt to gain 'mastery' over these abject reminders of the maternal body. In doing so, a defensive position is established within the organization in which the resurgence of abjected elements constantly threatens the prevailing order. I suggest this provides us with a provocative framework for understanding the government's current obsession with 'counting, control and calculation' (Power, 2004) within healthcare organizations, where the symbolic requirements of the 'audit culture', or the Law, are given precedence over feelings or the unarticulated drives of the body.

The following retrospective case study, drawing on my work as a psychotherapist and clinical supervisor within an IAPT service, attempts to illustrate some of the above dynamics. The material that I want to discuss is autoethnographical in nature and is reflective of my position at the time as a female senior clinician within the service. In this sense, I am a 'participant-observer', with both *one foot in and one foot out*' (Duncan & Diamond, 2011) of the organization, a position that enables me, as Parry and Boyle (2009) suggest, to 'uncover and illuminate the tacit and subaltern aspects of organisation, such as how actions which lead to negative or positive organisational outcomes actually play out' (p. 694).

Parry and Boyle (2009) also argue that a further advantage of organizational autoethnography is that it allows us to construct a richer, more informative understanding of organizational life, by 'connecting the micro and everyday and mundane aspects of organisational life with the broader political and strategic organisational agendas and practices' (p. 694). My decision to focus here on a single illustrative vignette demonstrating the way abjective dynamics are refracted in one particular organization thus aims to consider the complex interplay between unconscious dynamics, staff behaviour and the particular regulatory procedures to which both I and my colleagues were subject. In this respect, I hope a focus on the 'particular' offers the potential for understanding something of the 'universal' (Warnock, 1987), shedding light on the wider significance, function and mechanisms of abjection in public sector organizations.

Case example: improving access to psychological therapies

The 2008 launch of the UK government's IAPT programme sponsored an ambitious agenda of reform within primary care psychological services in the UK. While other chapters in this book will detail the political and economic background and evolution of IAPT, here I think it sufficient merely to point out that IAPT undoubtedly constitutes the single most significant state investment in mental health services since the inception of the NHS.

The IAPT model can be contextualized within an overall NPM framework within mental health services privileging increasingly standardized and regulated forms of practice within public sector services. Both inexperienced 'Psychological Wellbeing Practitioners' (PWPs) and trained cognitive-behavioural and other psychotherapists are required to undertake a battery of standardized diagnostic, assessment and treatment protocols, including multiple clinical measures at every contact with a client. They receive frequent case management in order to review their caseload and clinical outcomes and are required to evidence increasingly high activity and clinical outcome targets. Managers and service leads too are required to participate in similar regulatory mechanisms and to defend service activity and clinical outcomes to a centralized administration.

In the particular IAPT service in which I was employed, a large number of PWPs and cognitive-behavioural therapists were complemented by a small number of part-time psychotherapists offering short-term interventions and counselling for individuals referred for anxiety and depression. In line with our IAPT colleagues, my psychotherapist colleagues and I had recently been required to use the full IAPT dataset and software systems for recording clinical activity and outcome measures for each patient session. In addition, a decision was taken by senior management to expand psychotherapy provision to include several trainees who needed to gain clinical experience and practice hours for their professional accreditation. As their clinical supervisor, I was asked to ensure that these trainees complied with the IAPT data collection requirements, inputting their activity and clinical measures onto the same software system used by all practitioners in the service. The software system involved filling in each patient's demographic details, selecting a preliminary psychiatric diagnosis from a drop-down list and completing several sets of on-line clinical measures to be undertaken each time the client was seen.

During a clinical supervision session which I was facilitating, it was clear to me that one member of my group of three trainees appeared upset and agitated and needed to be heard as a matter of priority. She told the group that she had seen a patient the previous week and had been very worried that this young woman she had been working with had walked out of the session after 20 minutes. This patient had been referred for help with what the referring doctor had termed 'severe depression' following a recent termination and was finding it difficult to talk about her feelings of guilt, self-loathing and shame. At the start of the session, my trainee said she had persuaded her to complete the various clinical measures required by the service as she had been concerned at the patient's obviously depressed mood. After sullenly filling in the forms, her patient thereafter spent the session mainly in silence, remaining hunched in her coat with her chin tucked into the collar, tears continuously pouring down her face and her nose running. My trainee said that she had found this frank and uninhibited display of continual misery very difficult to bear: 'She had snot all over her face' she exclaimed, 'her collar was sodden; it was just . . . revolting!' The patient had largely ignored my trainee's efforts to engage her and seemed to be utterly sunk in a mood of rage alternating with apathy. Eventually, she had stood up and said that she couldn't put up with it anymore, and strode out of the room. My trainee said that she had felt 'completely paralysed', unable to think and was left feeling very worried indeed about her client. It transpired that during the week, she had found herself becoming increasingly uncomfortable, guilty and concerned at this young woman's psychological plight, and it had become apparent to her that she was spending quite a lot of time thinking about this young woman, something, she said, she was not used to doing.

She then said that a few days after the session she had been discussing the case with a senior cognitive-behavioural therapist in the service. It seemed to me, hearing my trainee's story at this point, that this very experienced (male) colleague of mine clearly felt that my trainee's anxiety was not justified by her patient's presentation and had tried to help her think more calmly about the case. He had asked to see the clinical measures that the trainee had taken from this young woman; and on finding that these were relatively low, said to her that there wasn't really any need to be too anxious, the patient was clearly showing sub-clinical scores, so she could not be held accountable were any risk issues to arise before the next session. In the group, my trainee said that she had felt partially reassured by this and then spoke at length, and with some tears of her own, about her unaccustomed feelings of disgust and repulsion at her patient's uncontrollable distress.

In fact, this colleague had spoken to me during the week about the incident, and it had been clear to me that he had become somewhat irritated with my trainee's request for help. Indeed, after a while he admitted that, although he had initially been pleased to talk to her, he couldn't really manage what he called 'all this anxiety'. He had work of his own to do and said that he had been feeling under considerable pressure to complete all his own data collection requirements in order to achieve his weekly targets. He spoke about the 'real requirements' of the service and suggested to me, politely but impatiently, that postgraduate psychotherapy trainees ought to be able to contain themselves better. 'They don't just want spoon-feeding,' he finally remarked, rather brusquely, 'they really want breastfeeding. It's not up to us to do that!' Somewhat taken aback at this rather vivid statement, I lamely tried to defend my trainee while struggling with a sudden mixture of anger, helplessness and what I later realized was a strong feeling of shame in myself; but it was to no avail. During the following week the clinical lead of the service asked me to ensure that my trainees did not request any further meetings with cognitive-behavioural therapists as this would reduce the time they needed to meet their increased activity targets.

Discussion

The conversation with my colleague had left me feeling confused, humiliated and angry, not just by the apparent relegation of my trainee to the status of demanding infant, but also, by extension, by my demotion to what I felt was some kind of nursemaid. Indeed, it is possible to understand my feelings of shame as a possible phenomenological index of the abjective dynamics at work here, arising in the face of a phallogocentric symbolic order dismissing the maternal, caring role as unnecessary to the 'real requirements' of the service. I certainly felt an underlying unease – and subsequently, as I admitted in supervision, outright anger – about the overt privileging of targets and data-collection, which I felt were the only aspects of clinical work recognized and acknowledged within the service. In part, my anger rested on an awareness of an already-present, deeply entrenched tension in the service between those whose training and theoretical orientation (cognitive-behavioural) favoured the IAPT culture and its emphasis on 'evidence-based clinical outcomes' (on which future funding depended), and those, like myself and my psychotherapist colleagues, whose theoretical interests (psychoanalytic) were more critical of such positivist epistemologies and praxes. In this sense, it can be seen that I had already positioned myself on one side of a fissure within the organization constituted along theoretical, clinical and, indeed, as the discussion with my colleague suggests, gendered lines; a split that my trainee and I were now struggling to manage.

Splitting, of course, is a familiar Kleinian term, pointing to the difficulty of integrating or reconciling ambivalent feelings. A traditional Kleinian reading of the above episode might also draw on Bion's (1962) notion of the 'container-contained', emphasising my trainee's difficulty in containing and managing her patient's feelings of anger and grief. Such an analysis might explore the way in which these feelings are subsequently split off and projected on to my colleague who then admits he cannot contain 'all this anxiety'. But I think a Kristevan reading helps us to focus on something occurring within the organization that cannot and will not be contained. The notion of breastfeeding is not only maternal, feminine: it is abject, a messy, leaky business involving the exchange of body fluids. My colleague's reaction suggests that he feels it is not up to him, either as a man or a clinician, to provide such intimate care for my trainee: rather, the more ordered, symbolic activity of clinical and diagnostic measures is invoked as a means of understanding and managing both the client's and the trainee's distress. More, the intimacy and blurring of boundaries implied in the notion of breastfeeding as metaphor for maternal, emotional care is contrasted with the need for more legitimate, 'real requirements' of 'data collection', something that is privileged within the organizational structure. 'A representative of the paternal function takes the place of the good maternal object that is wanting', writes Kristeva (1982). 'There is language instead of the good breast. Discourse is being substituted for maternal care' (p. 45). I suggest this opposition creates a continual movement or dynamic in the organization between the revulsion entailed by engaging in messy emotional contact ('breastfeeding') and the desire to undertake the more ordered, symbolic activities required of the organization. Indeed, the former could be said to mock the latter, threatening to subvert or sabotage the Law ('it's not up to us to do that!'). It was this dynamic that seemed to be exemplified by my trainee's inability to manage the distress and vulnerability of her patient who, silent and tearful, presented her with an experience of vulnerability and utter abjection for which the symbolic discourse of the service – its clinical measures – appeared radically insufficient. Indeed, the patient's presenting problem – the termination of an unwanted baby

– could be seen as paradigmatic of abjection itself: the violent expulsion of unwanted parts of the self, which are now threatening to return in her unspoken feelings of depression, rage and guilt.

In this case example, I suggest we can distinguish some of the ways in which a mental health service may confer abjection on staff and those they care for: first, by a process of psychiatric classification ('depression') that interpellates[3] the individual into a medical discourse, which thereafter defines his or her problem and determines what is deemed to be the appropriate kind of treatment for the diagnostic categories it generates; second, by subjecting managers and clinicians to increasing surveillance via clinical governance systems that regulate, evaluate and legitimate clinical activity and outcomes (the 'real requirements' of the service); and third, by the continual articulation, demarcation and extension of boundaries, rules and protocols within the service which define and proscribe 'the Law' – that is, what is or is not permitted to occur within the organization, between staff and within psychological treatment ('it's not up to us to do that!'). All these processes are clearly located within the Symbolic order, where the materiality and the corporeality of mental illness and psychological distress is specified, tabulated, diagnosed and otherwise situated within a phallogocentric discourse that exiles the emotional, messy – and maternal – aspects of caregiving. This in turn defends the organization against the 'monstrous' psychological fragility of individuals referred to the service as well as the feelings of staff who provide care for them. Of course, where society constructs caregiving as *necessarily* maternally oriented, there is a peculiar paradox between the explicit aims of a service to provide care for the mentally ill and the government-sponsored policies and protocols generating organizational dynamics, instrumental behaviour and clinical practice that serve to regulate, disavow and abject the very care such services are mandated by the public to provide. This in turn highlights a fundamental conflict between the explicit, rational aims of state-funded mental health provision and the unconscious, ambiguous and contradictory psychic mechanisms underpinning their implementation.

States of abjection

The above scenario offers us some insight into Fotaki's (2010) illuminating thoughts about 'why government policies fail so often'. Fotaki (2010) articulates the imaginary and phantasmatic basis of many UK government health policies, including the pursuit of '*Choice For All*', suggesting that such policies offer

> a stark testimony of the impossibility of realizing the policy objectives it proclaims, despite or perhaps because of its universalistic (and omnipotent) aspirations. . . . The attempt to attain the fantasy of the impossible can also explain policy recycling and repetition of the same ideas, despite many documented failures.
>
> *(p. 9)*

A central tenet of the IAPT programme has been to 'improve not only the health and well-being of the population, but also to promote social inclusion and improve economic productivity' (DoH, 2007, p. 4). Certainly, the politically ambitious scale of the IAPT mental health programme currently being marketed to the public with its promise of equal access to therapy for all and the notion that this will sponsor social inclusion and improved economic prosperity at a time of unprecedented global austerity may be regarded as aspirational at best, since such an agenda appears to be founded on the omnipotent and imaginary illusion of total unity, satisfaction and social harmony. Indeed, Fotaki (2010) argues on this basis that some government policies are prone to 'capture' by certain political groups for their own ideological purposes. This is certainly a persuasive reading of the IAPT agenda, which unequivocally recasts contemporary social and economic problems – the 'shit-life syndrome' I identified at the start of this chapter – within the template of middle-class individualism.

I suggest that as these state-governed aspirational policies are implemented across mental health services in the UK, social and organizational defences, including the dynamics of abjection, reinforce the impossibility of success, thus condemning such policies and the praxes they dictate to failure. Indeed, the problematic effects of recent government targets on healthcare, education and other public services have generated an entire literature (e.g. Bevan & Hood, 2006; Clapham, 2010; Hoggett, 2006, 2010; Shore, 2010; Shore & Wright, 1999). Notions of 'playing tick-box games' (McGivern & Ferlie, 2007) or 'gaming behaviour' (Bevan & Hood, 2006) suggest, along with the conclusions of the Francis Report (2013), that performance measurement systems similar to those currently being deployed within IAPT services may actually be 'fatal remedies' (Sieber, 1981) whose unintended consequences undermine the very activity they seek to assess and quantify. Perhaps it is not too much to suggest that these policies act to formalize a process of abjection within mental health services, giving rise to the unconscious dynamics illustrated above. If so, this offers a new way to understand the self-sabotaging nature of NPM reforms designed to improve transparency in public sector services (McGivern & Fischer, 2011; Strathern, 2000; Tsoukas, 1997) and brings a fresh perspective to how this is played out between staff and patients in a service. Perhaps what the above case study most vividly demonstrates is how mental health policy, unconscious organizational dynamics and clinical practice intersect to confer, sustain and enact abjection in ways that undermine and destabilize an organization's primary caring role.

Conclusion

In this chapter, I propose Kristeva's concept of abjection as a useful alternative lens through which to examine unconscious dynamics and processes within mental health services in general and IAPT services in particular. I argue that the presence of the abject serves as a perpetual if unconscious reminder of the existence of the 'monstrous' other within the self and offers a view of the divided individual as perpetually engaged in the struggle to demarcate his or her subjectivity. Clinical work within mental health services thus entails a continual effort by the organization and its staff to work with and empathically respond to patients who evoke unrecognized feelings of disgust and fear and from whom they simultaneously seek to distance themselves.

I also suggest that the continual abjection of reminders of the 'messy' maternal body and semiotic drives within mental health services paradoxically undermines and subverts the very care these services set out to provide. This supports the view that the rationalist agenda of many public health policies ignores the unconscious, irrational motivations that underlie clinicians' behaviour and fails to recognize how these may both be influenced by and contribute to the defensive practices of the organization. This links to the wider perspective discussed by Fotaki (2010) who points out that the rationalist and realist epistemology of contemporary socio-economics fails to take account of the unrecognized, imaginary or phantasmatic basis of much public health policymaking and is one reason why such policies fail so often.

Finally, I suggest that Kristeva's (1982) notion of abjection sheds new light on the nature of the 'rituals of verification' (Power, 1997) characteristic of NPM's growing demand for transparency, accountability and governance within public sector services. In the context of an IAPT mental health service, I have argued that an understanding of abjection contributes to our theoretical understanding of contemporary social practices of quality assurance, audit and evaluation, which can now be recast as the organizational attempt to defend and uphold the Symbolic order, and the struggle to define and maintain an institutional frontier against the semiotic drives of the body. This in turn potentially illuminates and deepens our understanding of the 'tyranny of transparency' (Strathern, 2000) common in public sector services as well as the related problems associated with clinical practitioners' 'reactivity' to regulatory mechanisms, for example in medicine and psychotherapy (McGivern & Fischer, 2011).

Just as we cannot get rid of shit, so I suggest we cannot free ourselves from psychological distress and mental ill-health. As Shildrick (2002) suggests, these issues arouse huge anxiety in us at both individual and organizational levels because they bring us into unwilling contact with our own abjected vulnerability, our own 'monstrous' need, our own ineluctable lack or fragmentation within. Indeed, the development and evolution of the IAPT programme as a whole can be understood as one way in which those involved in planning, commissioning and managing public sector mental health services have perhaps unconsciously colluded to control, overwrite or subdue the abject in the interests of managing public anxiety arising at a time of unprecedented economic austerity. In this chapter I have attempted to outline some of the ways in which an understanding of such processes may offer a fertile, if provocative, area for future debate and research.

Notes

1   This chapter is an edited version of a paper published in *Organization Studies* (2013) *34*(9), 1277–1297, and is reproduced here by kind permission of the Senior Editor, Yiannis Gabriel. Clinical details in both versions of the paper have been substantially altered to protect confidentiality.
2   The Lacanian 'Real' is not synonymous with reality. Rather, it denotes a primordial state of nature from which we are forever separated by our entry into language. The Real is opposed to the Imaginary and lies outside the Symbolic order. Indeed, its resistance to symbolization is what lends the Real its traumatic and anxiety-provoking quality.
3   Interpellation is a concept associated with Louis Althusser (1971), who uses the term to describe how individual identity is constituted through pre-existing ideologies, institutions and discourses which 'hail' the subject into being via social interactions.

References

Althusser, L. (1971). Ideology and ideological state apparatuses. In L. Althusser (ed.), *Lenin and philosophy and other essays*. New York: Monthly Review Press.
Bevan, G. & Hood, C. (2006). What's measured is what matters: Targets and gaming in the English public health care system. *Public Administration*, 84(3), 517–38.
Bion, W. (1962). *Learning from experience*. London: Heinemann.
Butler, J. (2004). *Undoing gender*. New York: Routledge.
Clapham, M. (2010). The sarcophagus of practice. In L. King & C. Moutsou (eds), *Rethinking audit cultures: A critical look at evidence-based practice in psychotherapy and beyond* (pp. 47–59). Ross-on-Wye, UK: PCCS Books.
Cooper, A. & Lousada, J. (2005). *Borderline welfare. Feeling and fear of feeling in modern welfare*. Tavistock Clinic Series. London: Karnac Books.
Department of Health (2007). *Commissioning a brighter future: Improving access to psychological therapies. Positive practice guide*. London: Department of Health.
Duncan, C. & Diamond, M. (2011). One foot in, one foot out: The paradox of participant-observation. *Sixth international conference on interdisciplinary social sciences*, Harry Truman School of Public Affairs, University of Missouri, 11–13 July.
Fotaki, M. (2011). The sublime desire for knowledge (in academia): Sexuality at work in business and management schools in England. *British Journal of Management*, 22(1), 42–53.
Foucault, M. (1964). *Madness and civilization: A history of insanity in the age of reason*. London: Routledge.
Foucault, M. (2003). *Abnormal. Lectures at the College de France 1974–1975*. London: Verso.
Freud, S. (1919). *The uncanny*. In Standard Edition, XVll (pp. 217–56), trans. J. Strachey. London: Hogarth Press.
Gabriel, Y. & Carr, A. (2002). Organizations, management and psychoanalysis: An overview. *Journal of Managerial Psychology*, 17(5), 348–65.
Hinshelwood, R. D. (1994). The relevance of psychotherapy. *Psychoanalytic Psychotherapy*, 8, 283–94.
Hoggett, P. (2006). Pity, compassion, solidarity. In S. Clarke, P. Hoggett & S. Thompson (eds), *Emotion, politics and society* (pp. 145–61). Basingstoke, UK: Palgrave Macmillan.
Hoggett, P. (2010). Government and the perverse social defence. *British Journal of Psychotherapy*, 26, 202–12.
Holmes, D., Perron, A. & O'Byrne, P. (2006). Understanding disgust in nursing: Abjection, self and the other. *Research and Theory for Nursing Practice: An International Journal*, 20(4) 305–15.

Hopfl, H. (2008). Sacred heart: A comment on the heart of management. *Culture and Organization*, 14(3), 225–40.

Keenoy, T. & Oswick, C. (2004). Organizing textscapes. *Organization Studies*, 25(1), 135–42.

Klein, M. (1946). Notes on some schizoid mechanisms. *International Journal of Psychoanalysis*, 27, 99–110.

Kristeva, J. (1982). *Powers of horror: An essay on abjection.* New York: Columbia University Press.

Lacan, J. (1953). 'Some reflections on the ego'. *The International Journal of Psychoanalysis*, 34, 11–17.

McGivern, G. & Ferlie, E. (2007). Playing tick-box games: Interrelating defences in professional appraisal. *Human Relations*, 60, 1361–1385.

McGivern, G. & Fischer, M. (2011). Reactivity and reactions to regulatory transparency in medicine, psychotherapy and counselling. *Social Science and Medicine*, 74, 286–96.

McGivern, G., Fischer, M., Ferlie, E. & Exworthy, M. (2009). Statutory regulation and the future of professional practice in psychotherapy and counselling: Evidence from the field. *ESRC report.* London: King's College.

Menzies-Lyth, I. (1959). The functioning of social systems as a defence against anxiety. *Human Relations*, 13, 95–121.

Obholzer, A. (2003). Managing social anxieties in public sector organizations. In J. Reynolds, J. Henderson, J. Seden, J. Charlesworth & A. Bullman (eds), *The managing care reader* (pp. 281–8). London: Routledge.

Parry, K., & Boyle, M. (2009). Organizational autoethnography. In D. Buchanan & A. Bryman (eds), *The Sage handbook of organizational research methods* (pp. 690–702). London: Sage.

Power, M. (1997). *The audit society: Rituals of verification.* Oxford: Oxford University Press.

Power, M. (2004). Counting, control and calculation. Reflections on measuring and management. *Human Relations*, 56, 765–83.

Report of the Mid Staffordshire NHS Foundation Trust Public Inquiry (2013), Chaired by Robert Francis QC. February 2013. London: The Stationery Office.

Riad, S., Vaara, E. & Zhang, N. (2012). The intertextual production of international relations in mergers and acquisitions. *Organization Studies*, 33(1) 121–48.

Shildrick, M. (2002). *Embodying the monster.* London: Sage.

Shore, C. (2010). Audit culture and illiberal governance: Universities and the politics of accountability. In L. King & C. Moutsou (eds), *Rethinking audit cultures: A critical look at evidence-based practice in psychotherapy and beyond* (pp. 11–36). Ross-on-Wye, UK: PCCS Books.

Shore, C. & Wright, S. (1999). Audit culture and anthropology: Neoliberalism in British higher education. *Journal of the Royal Anthropological Institution*, 5, 557–75.

Sieber, S. (1981). *Fatal remedies: The ironies of social intervention.* New York: Plenum Press.

Strathern, M. (2000). The Tyranny of transparency. *British Educational Research Journal*, 26(3), 209–321.

Thomas, R. & Davies, A. (2005). Theorizing the micro-politics of resistance: New public management and managerial identities in the UK public services. *Organization Studies*, 26(5), 683–706.

Tiezte, S. (2003). Metaphors of the mother. In H. Hopfl & M. Kostera (eds), *Interpreting the maternal organisation* (pp. 63–78). London: Routledge.

Townley, B. (1994). *Reframing human resource management.* London: Sage.

Tsoukas, H. (1997). The tyranny of light. *Futures*, 29(9), 827–43.

Warnock, M. (1987). *Memory.* London: Faber and Faber.

7

IAPT AND THE IDEAL IMAGE

Jay Watts

'. . . In the name of psychological science we seek fulfilment.'

Foucault (1984a, p. 261)

'It is the very pursuit of happiness that thwarts happiness.'

Viktor Frankl (1985, p. 85)

It is 2006. You are an MP, part of a New Labour once adored, now subject to ridicule. Your leader Tony Blair is now a figure of fun. It is unclear if you will win the next election. Suddenly, *The Depression Report* lands on your desk. The first page tells you that 'one in six of the population suffers from depression or chronic anxiety disorder'. This report promises results. You read on:

> At least half of them could be cured at a cost of no more than £750 . . . For depression and anxiety make it difficult or impossible to work, and drive people onto Incapacity Benefits. We now have a million people on Incapacity Benefits because of mental illness – more than the total number of unemployed people receiving unemployment benefits. . . . Mental illness is now the biggest problem, and we know what to do about it. . . . But can we afford the £750 it costs to treat someone? The money which the government spends will pay itself. For someone on Incapacity Benefit costs us £750 a month in extra benefits and lost taxes. If the person works just one month more as a result of the treatment, the treatment pays for itself!
>
> *(Layard et al., 2006)*

The language is sterling, but the message is better. *Cure*, no less, and in such a way that the country will actually *save* money. And an implicit promise of a happier voter, a voter – perhaps – more likely to want to keep the government the same. Who could blame our hypothetical MP for feeling keen.

A personal experience of IAPT

I too read the *Depression Report* in 2006, but I was less convinced for I was already one year into my Improving Access to Psychological Therapies (IAPT) experience. When I first qualified, in 2005, I started a job in East London. Within days, I heard that the area was being put forward as one of two pilot sites for a new project called IAPT. Local clinicians were in two minds. Was this an opportunity for us, in the most economically deprived area in the country, to have an injection of funding first for once? Or was this initiative, based as it was on CBT, a pipe dream, introducing a model of therapy, based on norms which just did not fit with our deprived, diverse, local community? Over the coming years, I would attend round after round of consultations. Would it work, had it worked, couldn't we see it had worked? As evidence from the local pilot study was used to roll out the programme nationally, many of us became confused. Had our feedback not been considered – the exponential increase in new referrals to secondary services, the people who had been 'cured' but came back for more, the success stories, yes, but envy that was bubbling up between the old and new workforce. The version of IAPT that was being storied was one glossier and more evangelical than the reality.

My concern for the chasm between the image of IAPT and the actuality of IAPT has only increased over the years as I have supervised dozens of IAPT workers, listened to hour upon hour of tapes of IAPT sessions and heard the stories of patients who have been through IAPT. These experiences have all led me to believe that IAPT operates in a virtuality focusing on performativity and surveillance rather than real encounters between clinician and patient. I believe this can be a huge strain on IAPT clinicians and is the main reason that vast numbers of people referred to IAPT never successfully complete a treatment (e.g. McInnes, 2014).

Arguments for IAPT are presented as so commonsensical that to answer 'no' to the question 'Are you against improving access to psychological therapies?' seems ridiculous. Yet some times we need to trouble common sense, to listen to what does not quite fit, to wonder what becomes of those burnout workers, the hundreds of thousands – of referrals that disappear before receiving a 'successful' treatment (e.g. Griffiths, Foster, Steen & Pietroni, 2013). This chapter is about wondering what does not fit the image of IAPT and how the seeming gloss of its promises may actually increase the level of anguish in society.

The right treatment, the right choice

As I started to write this chapter, a flyer came through my letterbox, part of an initiative to sell online IAPT Cognitive Behavioural Therapy (CBT) to all Camden residents. It insists that *my* personality is worthy of attention – that I can have any sadness, anxiety, unhappiness that might get in the way of who I would want myself to be excised. It is an exciting option. The promise of finding out if I am sadder than I should be brings back echoes of quizzes in girls' magazines when I was a teenager – tantalising promises to answer the questions 'does he fancy you?', 'are you popular?' A chance to quantify exactly how I am doing, a promise to conquer sadness! Who wouldn't be tempted by such an idea? Yet at what cost?

To address these questions, we need to explore the treatment that is being proposed, CBT. Over the past 25 years, CBT has become the treatment of choice in England (Harvey, Watkins, Mansell & Shafran, 2004). There are many reasons for its dominance, but briefly it is cheaper than most therapies, highly marketable and fits well with the grand narrative of evidence-based medicine (House & Loewenthal, 2008). Unlike many psychotherapies, CBT has a model of psychic change which allows it to be tested through Randomised Controlled Trials (RCTs), the gold star of the NICE guidelines, which structure service provision in the UK (Slade & Priebe, 2001). CBT has come to replace older treatments such as family or psychodynamic therapy in the hearts and minds of commissioners and, increasingly, the public with young generations increasingly referring to it as a lifestyle option.

CBT is storied as 'forward looking' and 'positive'; not 'endless nor backward-looking' (The Depression Report, 2006, p. 1) as other therapies are caricatured. This is an inviting narrative, the forward, progressive narrative (good) implicitly opposed to a backwards (bad) one. These discursive moves to rubbish what was before and present CBT as exciting are necessary to engineer a position where CBT is picked as a treatment in an era of consumer choice. Consider this piece of prose:

> If you have depression or are worried you might have, you need good information to make the right choice about different kinds of help. This booklet tells you about the range of evidence-based talking therapies that are approved by the National Institute for Health and Clinical Excellence (NICE) for treating adults with depression. It aims to give you the information you need, help you *ask the right questions* and decide which therapy suits you. These therapies have been shown to be at least as effective in treating depression as flu vaccines are in preventing flu, beta-blockers in treating high blood pressure or surgery in removing cataracts – and they can be safer and more effective in the long term than prescribed drugs.
>
> *('Which Talking Therapy for Depression?' DoH, 2011, p. 1)*

Though the purpose of the leaflet is purposively to help the reader choose 'which talking therapy', the words explicitly and implicitly encourage the reader to ask the 'right questions' to make the 'right choice' consistent with the grand narrative of evidence-based medicine – a 'choice' storied as so commonsensical that it is akin to choice in physical medicine. Fluent in the grand narratives of evidence base and cost–benefit analysis, CBT is the 'right choice' for the era of New Public Management (Hood, 1991, p. 59), whereby 'market discipline has been applied to public bureaucracies through reforms which have attempted to increase competition'. NPM is the bureaucratic manifestation of neo-liberalism – the merger of liberal ideas with free-market economics that originated in the 1980s. CBT fits well in an era which combines a competitive, economic focus with an 'audit explosion' (Power, 1997). To understand why, we must first explore what CBT is like in IAPT and the experience of the IAPT worker.

Excision versus exploration

CBT is a set of techniques that focus on problems in the here-and-now (Harvey *et al.*, 2004). CBT aims to remove 'symptoms' or alter a patient's relation to them, and not look for their hidden meanings. CBT promises to allow us to cut out bits that do not fit with our 'ideal image' of ourselves. There is no unpacking of the 'ideal image' of what we should be, what is normal, what is desirable, and how it has been created from the remnants of our upbringing, our histories, the socio-political reality that we have been raised in. The emphasis is less on 'why' a problem emerged rather than 'how' an individual contributes to its 'maintenance' in their current thought patterns and beliefs.

CBT is focused on a 'case conceptualisation' or formulation. In IAPT services, as opposed to with CBT with more complex presentations like psychosis or so-called personality disorders (e.g. Morrison & Barratt, 2010), a case conceptualisation takes the form of tailoring the patient's experiences to a model of their designated problem which is set out in (quite literally) boxes and downloadable from the central governing IAPT organisation and organisations such as UCL's CORE unit. Problems are seen as a result of faulty reasoning or behaviours in the individual. In contrast, most other therapeutic approaches have attempted to contextualise distress, be they psychodynamic approaches which contexualise the symptom with the psychodynamics of competing mental systems, family therapies which entexture the system in wider systems, or feminist therapies which politicise and gender personally embodied distress. While the CBT literature pays lip service to the increased prevalence of distress in certain populations and increasingly, the importance of early trauma, such as bullying, in the origins of problems (e.g. Corrigan & Hull, 2014), clinical practice communicates something different. For though sometimes, nowadays, there may be a box in the formulation for 'early childhood experiences' where bullying or sexual abuse may be written, the focus of the work is not on acknowledging or working through these experiences. This communicates to the patient that the responsibility, now, is theirs.

Collorating with empiricism?

Though there is surface talk that CBT for common problems does not follow the medical model (e.g. Department of Health, 2011), the models for particular problems taught on IAPT training programmes are strangely familiar to anyone who knows the diagnostic system (i.e. specific phobias, panic disorder, social phobia,

OCD, PTSD, Generalised Anxiety Disorder and Health Anxiety and Body Dysmorphic Disorder). The use of problems akin to diagnostic categories gives an implicit impression that the faulty cognitions and behaviours are due to a disorder and that this provides an actual explanation as opposed to a mere label. This problematises the 'collaborative empiricism' between patient and therapist that is used in CBT to brand the approach, for the style of questioning is steeped in a presumption not just that this way of seeing the 'problem' is correct, but that this is a value neutral, invisible activity.

Most assessments are carried out on the telephone. The clinician's task is to assess risk and establish which 'problem' the patient has so they can be placed on the Psychological Wellbeing Practitioner's (PWP) or High Intensity Worker's (HI) waiting list (or stepped up to secondary care if need be). Thus a thorough psychological assessment is not carried out, nor does the question and answer protocol driven format allow a chance to listen to the patient's complaint. This may be an important defence against anxiety (e.g. Menzies-Lyth, 1959) for the overwhelmingly social causes of mental distress (e.g. World Health Organization, 2014) cannot be cured in IAPT's average of 3.94 sessions (Griffiths & Steen, 2013). Under such circumstances, we can understand, perhaps, the desire not to know.

The IAPT patient will then start treatment with a different clinician who will have been primed to which problem s/he is expected to work through from the assessment. Sessions last for up to half an hour for PWP workers, but many are just ten minutes in comparison with 50 minute session times within psychotherapy (e.g. Feltham & Horton, 2012). The pressure to meet session number deadlines means techniques must be taught as quickly as possible after a brief 'socialisation into the model' of CBT. The patient has already been primed into the idea that internal problems can be readdressed through changing faulty thinking or behaviours through the way assessment questions are formulated and the implicit messages about the model in referral information and leaflets. The extortionately high rates of drop outs at this stage suggest many vote against CBT with their feet; these drop outs are not seen as failures of CBT in the analysis of outcome data as presented by IAPT (McInnes, 2014).

Socialising or indoctrinating?

For those patients who remain, an 'agenda' is set at the start of each session, and the homework set at the previous session is discussed.[1] Agenda and homework setting are both storied as collaborative endeavours in the CBT literature. However, when supervising tapes of IAPT workers, it is clear that in the majority of cases clinicians suggest or steer patients to IAPT consistent goals such as applying for a job or going out in public. This is less because of malevolent intentions but because of the twin evils of a) lack of time so severe that procrastination of decision making is not just possible and the patient needs to be encouraged and b) socialisation into the idea that therapy is about *doing* things, getting somewhere, rather than listening. Thus, for the IAPT worker, it seems perfectly natural that homework tends to focus on either attempted 'behavioural change' or monitoring existing thoughts to replace them with alternatives rather than going on a march or painting. The resistance to this – implicit in the high rate of non-compliance with homework with 40 per cent not completing it (e.g. Schmidt & Woolaway-Bickel, 2000) – is attributed to faulty technique on behalf of the therapist who, we we will see, is perpetually monitored herself.

The majority of sessions are spent on 'eliciting key cognitions', 'eliciting and planning behaviours' and 'guided discovery'. The choice of words here is revealing. For example, 'eliciting' means to evoke or draw out with the assumption that we extract from someone what we know to already be there. This is an apt description of the CBT model because, for common problems such as the models of social anxiety and others, the practitioners do purport to know the main fault in cognitions and behaviours to draw out. The therapist and patient need to go through a performance of finding this out, as if it were not already predetermined, before applying a set of 'change methods' or techniques to fine tune the muscle of the human machine. Thus, techniques are applied to individual subjectivity initially from outside, which the individual is encouraged to absorb, creating new subjectivities at the cost of what the symptom was, perhaps, trying to tell us. Darian Leader has compared this facet of CBT to the Maoist Cultural revolution in China, where depression was reframed as due to faulty thinking rather than the trauma of displacement or poverty (Leader, 2008). Certainly, the 'technologies of the self' that the CBT patient is taught carries echoes of Foucault's 'disciplinary power' (e.g. Foucault, 1984b) where the state uses subtle power to mould its subjects into acquiescence. Nikolas Rose (1990) has argued that this modern 'governmentality' of selfhood 'conducts the conduct' of citizens in line with a neo-liberal ideology which construes the self as a psy self-improvement project for which the state has minimal responsibilities. This makes listening to IAPT tapes sound like listening to torture – but what I hear is patients giving up what they want to talk about for what the IAPT worker wants to, needs to, introduce. They do this often for what psychoanalysts might call 'transference love' (Freud, 1958); the power of the relationship to make us suggestive to what the other would have us be may sound far-fetched, but it is perhaps the only explanation for why all therapies, whatever the model, however different the epistemology, work equally well (e.g. Norcross & Lambert, 2011).

Second-wave versus third-wave CBTs

Defenders of CBT argue critics do not know what contemporary CBT is like (e.g. Samuels & Veale, 2009), confusing so-called 'second wave' CBTs, which focus more on trying to control or alter thoughts, with 'third-wave' CBTs, which focus more on challenging emotional avoidance and troubling people's habit of taking thoughts seriously. However, though it is true that third-wave CBTs use the relationship more (e.g. Churchill *et al.*, 2013), the type of CBT practices in IAPT is overwhelmingly second-wave as this is easier and quicker to teach through guided bibliotherapy and short-term change techniques. As CBT in IAPT is so time squeezed, there is no space to question these implicit values. Such a CBT is more akin to a fitness programme for the mind, an analogy explicitly used (IAPT, 2011). The CBT patient in IAPT services, devoid of space to explore his or her own values to angle towards must take in lieu the ready-made norms provided by the state.

The CBT practised by PWPs is not akin to the more sophisticated therapy offered by HIs or in secondary services – PWPs are not therapists, we hear. Yet the headlines and policy documents group PWPs as 'the new workforce of therapists' (IAPT, 2011) blurring the loss of what even the IAPT and CBT communities recognise as a different experience. The need in a short period of time to provide a solution dictates the incorporation of a set of ideas about the cause of problems imposed from outside into the subjectivities of patients. We find this phenomenon equally with the new treatments that are slowly beginning to be available in IAPT – Dynamic Interpersonal Therapy (Lemma, Target & Fonagy, 2011) and Behavioural Couples Therapy for Depression (e.g. Bodenmann et al., 2008). These therapies – from psychodynamic and couples therapy traditions – ignore the deconstructionist elements of these modalities for a practice that shores up defences and normalises the subjectivities of those with symptoms trying to speak. Hence it is not just CBT that falls into the remit of what Langs (1979) called a 'lie therapy'; it is the neo-liberal insistence on the proceduralisation of practice, the surveillance of workers and the forces of the market which impose on the patient a framework of who they are and how, from now on, they must act.

I hope that I have begun to trace how, though there are specifics to CBT which make it complicit with neo-liberal ideology, the very structure of IAPT worsens this tenfold. I now turn to the position of the IAPT worker – a clinician under more pressure, monitoring and surveillance than any talking therapist in history – and the socialisation into one way of seeing the human psyche which IAPT training consists of.

Workability as a good outcome

> As a general rule what we find today is that the further removed observers (i.e. managers, policy makers, politicians) are from the reality of the front-line the more they are likely to be taken in by the illusion they themselves have been instrumental in creating.
>
> *Hoggett (2010, p. 61)*

Most IAPT teams consist of a manager, senior supervising clinicians (most often Clinical or Counselling Psychologists), High Intensity Workers, Psychological Wellbeing Practitioners and Employment Advisers tasked with helping attendees get back into employment. The presence of Employment Advisors is crucial to IAPT, for it is the cost–benefit reduction for society which was used to justify initial funding (Draper, 2006). Many critiques of IAPT have examined the problems with such analyses, based as they are on cure rather than 'reliable recovery', which more likely sees many 'successful patients' still falling within diagnostic criteria (e.g., Department of Health, 2010). Here, I focus more on the insidious effect their presence has on how 'therapy' is practised. Let us start with an example from one IAPT's website 'Help to Get and Stay in Work' (2010):

> Many of our treatments will look at ways of helping you get a job, or secure a job you already have. We know that many of the symptoms of depression and anxiety make being in work difficult, so we will work with you to manage these negative effects.

This discourse, the physical presence of the employment worker in meetings, and collection of outcome data on employability and benefits all serve to indoctrinate the IAPT worker into an ideal of what 'cure' should look like. The link between IAPT and workability was made explicitly by politicians in charge of funding the initiative. For example:

> Imagine there was a new policy, sitting on a shelf somewhere, that could, at surprisingly low cost, and in just a matter of months, transform millions of people's lives. Imagine . . . it would make people more employable and better parents, thereby increasing productivity, cutting the benefits bill and reducing antisocial behaviour. New Labour Advisor Derek Draper.
> *(Draper, 2006)*

The unexplored assumption is that health = work = good. Accordingly, homework tasks frequently linked to increasing workability by sending in an application or attending a job centre. The patient receives a clear message that the 'invisible standard' is that of a working, compliant person whose sadness is not so devastating, his anger not so forceful as to bother others. This presumption of what a good outcome is differs dramatically from the traditional ethics of a psychotherapy where a good outcome cannot be named (e.g. House & Loewenthal, 2008) and quite often takes the form of a patient abandoning introjected societal norms to pursue a passion. For example, a patient might leave a career as a bank clerk – a good, safe career desire by a parent – for the much desired instability of being a freelance artist. Such a psychotherapy is not as consistent with the neo-liberal agenda, the world of 'rights and responsibilities', which the modern subject is socialised into. The association of workability with changing faulty cognitions rather than social position serves to equate worklessness with what Scanlon and Adlam (2010) call 'worthlessness'. The emergence of psy-welfare thus provides a way for politicians to blame the individual as opposed to their policies without appearing to point blame. This psychologisation of fault is left with the patient, with the IAPT worker acting as an unassuming go-between for the state to communicate this message to the individual.

The new therapists who are not therapists

PWPs are 61 per cent of the 'new workforce' that is central to IAPT's endeavour (IAPT, 2011) and hold an even higher percentage of the caseload as HIs see far fewer patients. In IAPT propaganda – policy document, government announcements, newspaper headlines – they are constantly included in the numbers as new therapists. Yet PWPs are explicitly and continuously told they are not therapists and do not carry out therapy. The best practice guidelines for PWPs focus on a core skill: *not* to 'Carry out "medium intensity" therapy' or 'drift from using evidence-based low-intensity principles like CBT self-help resources aimed at step two, into doing "therapy"' (IAPT, 2011). Rather:

> A PWP's professional relationship with patients can be likened to a CBT self-help 'coach' role, such as an athletics coach or a personal fitness trainer. If people go to the gym or play sports, fitness trainers do not do the actual physical work of getting them fit. That is up to the individual. However, the trainer will help devise a fitness plan, monitor a person's progress and keep encouraging them when the going gets tough. A PWP will act in the same way.
>
> *(Psychological Wellbeing Practitioners: Best Practice Guidelines.*
> *IAPT, 2011, p. 5)*

PWP workers are thus therapists when it is politically expedient only. This blurriness has real consequences as the existence of IAPT's new workforce has been used to convince commissioners that therapy can be carried out by a cheaper workforce leading to the deletion of qualified posts. Further, GPs and the public are given the impression patients are getting 'psychological therapies' rather than guided self-help. This distinction is not merely academic, for if someone has had something once, they are less likely to be offered or seek it again. The therapy box has been, seemingly, ticked.

PWP training consists of a one year course with four days supervised practice; HIs receive two days' training a week for a year with three days supervised practice. During training, PWPs hold an average annual caseload of 170 patients in comparison with psychotherapy trainees who will see a handful of training cases over three or four years. The training for PWPs tends to be carried out by senior professionals, such as clinical psychologists, nearly all of whom have never worked by telephone, carried out guided self-help or had such time constraints on their work. This allows trainers to maintain and teach an idealised version of IAPT treatment for a patient wholly imagined. It is the workers who face the reality on the ground:

> My training was poor and did not prepare me well for seeing 'actual' people with 'real' problems that cannot be solved with some insincere empathy and a problem statement! I saw people with sometimes a 20 or 30+ year history

of mental health difficulties all of which impact on them in the here and now and very little of which I could actually, realistically help with. All of our therapy practice was done through role plays with each other and then trained actors.

PWP Worker (Internet Forum)

I've so often witnessed HI CBT trainees bouncing back cases to the wait-list because the course has deemed them 'not a suitable training case'. When 80 per cent of your wait-list are 'not a suitable training case,' something is going very wrong in what you are training people to do. In contrast, placement people from other trainings seem to take on a far wider selection of cases.

HI (Internet Forum)

Some IAPT workers enjoy their work of course – it has given a huge number of people entry level positions in an area that enjoys increasing cultural authority. Yet the huge caseloads place a huge strain on PWPs. This is not something that those in power wish to hear:

There is no emphasis on looking after you as an individual with a potentially ridiculous caseload and high stress levels due to the complex nature of the people you are asked to see (don't be fooled by the mild to moderate labels you might have heard!) (my caseload at one point was 75+) in PWP supervision – it is literally a numbers exercise e.g. how many people are you carrying, their difficulty and what you are going to do to help them. When I raised concerns that I was stressed I more or less got told to 'put up and shut up'.

PWP Worker (Internet Forum)

Proceduralism versus the personal

The simplicity of the prototypical patient trainees are taught about and the perceived commonality of patients in the various groups serves an important function – to decrease interest in the lived experience and reality of the patient once the trainee is in a service setting:

I found the role-plays outside the Observed Clinical Structured Exam fairly useful if only because other trainees are likely to get bored and add in complicated stuff just to stay interested.

PWP Worker (Internet Forum)

This proceduralism is an important defence if one is being asked to encounter 250 patients a year (IAPT, 2011).

Apart from caseload, the most pernicious pressure on IAPT workers is to gain outcome measures for each session. During training, workers are sold into the excitement of producing the largest database on wellbeing in history. There is no attention paid to the problematic nature of evidence-base in mental health (e.g. Slade & Priebe, 2001) nor the effects the taking of routine outcomes have on human subjectivity. For, being asked to score oneself on criteria sets up an 'invisible standard' of how one should be thinking or feeling. This process is made worse in IAPT for the outcome measures in the dataset – the PHQ-9 and GAD-7 – only ask questions about the patient's internal state. This choice of outcome measures solidifies the individualisation of distress. Other choices were available, for example, if the minimum data set used is an 'empowerment scale' (e.g. Rogers, Chamberlin, Ellison & Crean, 1997), sub scales such as 'righteous anger', 'power, and 'community activism' would be seen as central to the direct treatment for the elimination of anxiety one finds in the GAD-7. Thus messages sent to the patient about good wellbeing are shaped by the outcome messages used. Resistance often takes the part of parapraxes on behalf of the patient or worker, which, untheorised in the CBT model, go unnoted.

> Because, quite often, people don't come for their last session, you know, their therapy is completed and we weren't aware that the last time we saw them was going to be the last session. That's been fairly disappointing. I think a lot of the time the therapist, including me, forgets them.
>
> *HI worker (cited in Griffiths et al., 2013, p. 46)*

The way suggestion can steer what is said is acknowledged though.

> You can easily do it: 'Oh you're much better now, aren't you – I'm sure that's a six . . . I think you've been doing much better this week, don't you think that's a two'?
>
> *Commissioner (cited in Griffiths et al., 2013, p. 27)*

There is little real chance to escape the pernicious shaping of outcome measures, for they are required to be reviewed for each patient every four weeks in weekly case management supervision and tapes supervised for adherence to the model. Given the limits of supervisory time, looking at the numbers takes the place of listening to what the patient has said or the worker has experienced.

Performativity

The pressure to be able to perform effectiveness, rather than actually be effective, has increased since the introduction of 'Payment by Results' (Appleby & Jobanputra, 2004) and 'Any Qualified Provider' (Reynolds & McKee, 2012), whereby the contract for local IAPT service is given based on a competitive, bidding process. Thus we hear from one manager:

Does everyone miraculously get healed in week 11 because payment stops in week 12 . . . or week six for the low tariff? I remember many events, where I was suspicious of the motivations of some of the clinicians, and I was harangued for such prejudice and you know, no clinician would ever extend a session beyond its natural clinical usefulness. Incentives kick in, and the need to pay the mortgage.

IAPT Manager (cited in Griffiths et al., 2013, p. 22)

There are, as one commissioner told me recently, 'incentives for the data not to be accurate', leaving some patients alienated between how they seem to have progressed and their actual lived experience. No wonder, then, that so many IAPT workers intend to leave, with a quarter of workers leaving in the first three years (source North West IAPT programme).[2] But leave for where?

The dominance of the mantra 'what is recordable and measurable is good' has had ripple effects on service organisations and other professions. Therapists from other modalities, often with decades of experience, have found themselves considered an expensive, often expendable luxury in comparison with IAPT workers. This 'new workforce' of 'competent professionals' carries in its discourse an implicit criticism of other therapies as being old and incompetent. Yet such 'old and incompetent' clinicians must also bear the patients whose symptoms cannot be boxed into the IAPT symptom, often those with the most chaotic lives and intransigent symptoms. The old workforce must also bear considerable envy for their higher wages, their seeming capacity to work with fewer patients, and often their capacity to contain the anxiety of another subjectivity and real madness. Moreover concern about IAPT from outsiders and the 'old workforce', such as the authors in this book, is rubbished for being anti-progressive and old-fashioned; the venom here perhaps carries with it the lopsided fear that perhaps the project is problematic after all. Yet it is difficult to find space to resist when formally radical community organisations such as MIND have rebranded themselves as excellent organisations for IAPT tenders, and training courses find their accreditations contingent on teaching IAPT curriculums. Under such pressure, it can be reassuring for the 'new workforce' to return to the rhetorical certitude of the IAPT literature with its seeming promises of cure, recovery, the new and a few juicy vignettes of success to lure one in. In anxious times, the rhetoric of conviction is especially appealing.

A patient's experience

The fuel that has made me write this chapter is the experience of patients whose stories are not represented in the ever so short glossy vignettes one finds in IAPT leaflets. I would like to present one, in brief.

A few months ago, I received a call from a woman I will call Rachel who[3] I had seen for a few sessions prior to her move to University a couple of years before. Rachel was on a bridge, about to jump. I said I was here to listen to her, made sure she got to a safe place, then asked her what had happened. She was in a relationship with a man, John, who consistently and sadistically emotionally abused her to the extent that she would rip at her hair and cower in the corner. He had cut her off from her friends, family and former life. The relationship had been good until he cheated, whereafter he projected all his hate feeling like his cheating onto Rachel. He said she was nothing, ugly, most likely infertile, that no one would marry her, ever want her, she was disgusting. This he said: 'one centimetre' from her face, sometimes with his hand clasped around her throat. Such violence repeated something of Rachel's brother's rage at her, a rage that emerged quite suddenly when she started puberty, a rage taken out at her quite unmediated by any parental intervention. After weeks of abuse, Rachel would sometimes crack and scream or throw things at John or shout in a desperate bid to get him to give her some space. This allowed him a new line of attack – to say that she was mad, and 'had an anger management problem', an accusation he repeated hundreds of times. After some months of this attack, desperate to appease him, Rachel agreed she had a problem and went to her GP. She was referred to IAPT and took this fact as a present to John – it was she who had the problem, not him, not his infidelity, not his rage. When I spoke to her on the bridge, it was a week since her assessment with IAPT. The assessor had given her no space to talk, but seen 'anger problems' on the GP's letter and seen this as a problem within Rachel, following a pro-forma and asking a series of predesigned questions without finding out anything about her context. At one point, the question 'Had she ever hit anyone', Rachel answered 'yes' and was told immediately she was too serious a case for IAPT, that domestic abuse to men was 'just as bad as to a woman', and that the worker was duty bound to call the police. A week later not only was John using this encounter as evidence he was right and escalated his violence, but the promise the police would be involved – for the wrong partner, but still an action – had not materialised. There was nothing left for Rachel but to jump, except the faint memory of an encounter a long time before where she had been asked to speak freely, an activity she would start again as a step to disentangle the discourses of individualised pathology which threatened her life.

Rachel's unconscious desire in going to the GP was perhaps a flailing attempt to seek the input, help and intervention that mum had never managed between her and her brother. The presumption of what is going on once a key signifier – 'anger', 'sadness', 'anxiety' – in IAPT stops this being heard. As Rachel said later 'even the most basic, simple questioning of why I was angry would have led to me talking about John'. Rachel's case would not come across as a failure of IAPT as it is performed currently. She must be part of a statistic somewhere of people 'not suitable for IAPT', an extra digit in an assessor's contact figures for that week. Yet the contact was near fatal. We cannot know how John came across the idea of 'anger management' as a way to attack her, nor what would have happened had she not had an experience of therapy once before. However what we can tell from her experience – for I know it is not exceptional – is that proceduralism stops even basic relational contact between a mental health practitioner and someone in anguish.

The fault for this cannot be laid at the door of any particular worker, for structurally IAPT does not allow them the time to wonder why and what. The IAPT worker is the most scrutinised clinical worker in history – constantly monitored for their clinical work adherence to the CBT model, supervised on a case-by-case basis by supervisors needing to see progress in outcomes, watched by managers to ensure they reach the fewest number of contact hours with the most number of patients to meet service outcomes. The sheer volume of checklists, let alone the caseload, reminds us of Menzies-Lyth's (1959) work on how depersonalisation, categorisation and denial of the significance of the individual are used to defend against the anxiety of death, despair, the body and fragility. Checking off symptoms is an effective way to not be with them, a collaboration that may serve the interests of both therapist and patient. This 'fetishisation of bureaucracy' in the NHS (Rizq, 2012) is part of a wider rise in 'audit culture' (Power, 1999) as numbers become a safer site of worship than professions or even science. The worship of 'evidence' at this moment of history, unfortunately, forecloses the fact that numbers are only collected specific to particular ideologies and can be massaged to particular ends. Thus the 'auditable surface' (Cummins, 2002) is a compelling way to make things *seem* a certain way, but the reality will be different. As Terkel (1978) noted in an early study on the effects of performance target, 'developing the arts of impression management' becomes the key defence. It is one that stops pain being listened to and the meaning of symptoms heard.

Shaping minds

IAPT gives to its patients 'techniques of the self' (Foucault, 1974) to make them govern themselves with the eaten-in norms that make the state run smoothly. The rolling out of CBT and IAPT are heightened examples of a relatively new idea – that the self is a project which can be moulded and chipped away at so as to become attractive to the market. Such ideas have been building since the self-help slogans of actualisation began to enter the cultural landscape in the 1970s (e.g. Lasch, 1979). IAPT promotes these ideas as demands on the individual. Thus, though the title of Lord Layard's latest book 'Thrive' is presumably supposed to be an invitation, it also comes across as an edict. We can and must erase parts of our personality which do not sell well in the modern market place of the self, and CBT – the implication goes – can help us do that. The promise that this is possible, that we can 'cure' depression and anxiety, only fuels the lack we feel in comparison with the images of perfection on our computer screens and in our magazines. This lack in itself creates what is called mental illness. The discourse around CBT implies that we can alter bits of the self that we do not like in the ultimate self-fashioning project. If the only options for understanding not thriving are moral failure or mental illness, then most will choose the latter. Even more so as the idea of mental illness can now be used to situate the self within an arc of recovery, a transformative narrative almost ubiquitous now in biographies, reality TV shows or successful blogs. The insistence that common feelings, such as sadness and depression, can be cured is highly specific to our time and reflects what Rimke and Brock (2011) have called 'the shrinking spectrum of normalcy'. As Nikolas Rose (1990) traces out in *Governing the Soul*, the psyche has traditionally been seen as a site of a structurally unwinnable war between passion and reason, desire and society. The promises of happiness and wellbeing that IAPT propounds and inserts into our letterboxes constitutes an ever more impossible-to-reach 'ego ideal' or 'image of the perfect self towards which the ego should aspire' (Chasseguet-Smirgel, 1975). The chasm between this ego ideal and our lived reality only increases the level of anguish and pain in our communities.

This finding is clear from an exploration of what happens when IAPT is introduced into an area. It is perhaps for this reason that the NHS mental health services have been subject to unprecedented service redesign since IAPT was launched in 2005. In East London, the first two years of IAPT produced a substantial increase in referrals to secondary services. This was storied as due to the uncovering of 'hidden populations' of those in anguish who had suffered in silence beforehand and thus been excluded from analysis of the pilot site results. When four years after the introduction of IAPT, this phenomenon refused to cease, it became clear that IAPT was making people question their own mental health and doubt their capacity to cope. It made people demand more of themselves, and more of the NHS. We found our secondary care service redesigned once the reality of the effect of IAPT on secondary care became apparent – our service served the same function but was relabelled so that, theoretically, it was a new service. Thus, before and after comparisons could no longer be made. Similar smoke and mirrors are being used up and down the country to mask the reality of managed care.

There is a virtual reality to welfare governance today, an 'as if' character of achievement with the fetishisation of number crunching giving an image of success increasingly blurry with what is actually happening on the ground. IAPT makes it appear 'as if' problems were internally produced – as if they could be separate and distinct from social conditions and opportunities despite an international evidence base that this is not the case (WHO, 2014). The powerful get something from this cultural shift. Politicians get a way to appear to help problems their policies have helped create. GPs get to feel they are offering something to get the repeat attendees with no real physical symptom to go away. Psy staff get more prestige and cultural authority. Yet it is impossible to maintain a 'thick skin'(Cooper & Lousada, 2005; Hoggett, 2010) between how numbers perform according to IAPT and the lived experience of so many whose referral led to nothing or who are charged with providing a treatment to those whose reality does not meet the textbook. We cannot, should not, allow their voices to go unheard.

Notes

1   All the words in quotations in the following section come from the main adherence scale to CBT (CTS-R – Blackburn *et al.*, 2001). They are the core competencies for CBT.
2   This scuppers IAPT's cost projections, which are based on the presumption that IAPT workers, once trained, would stay.

3   This former client – who I have called 'Rachel' – has given written consent for her experience to be used. Nonetheless, I have anonymised potentially identifying features of the case.

References

Appleby, J. & Jobanputra, R. (2004). Payment by results. *New Economy*, 11(4), 195–200.

Blackburn, I. M., James, I. A., Milne, D. L., Baker, C., Standart, S., Garland, A. & Reichelt, F. K. (2001). The revised cognitive therapy scale (CTS-R): Psychometric properties. *Behavioural and Cognitive Psychotherapy*, 29(4), 431–46.

Bodenmann, G., Plancherel, B., Beach, S. R., Widmer, K., Gabriel, B., Meuwly, N., Charvoz, L., Hautzinger, M. & Schramm, E. (2008). Effects of coping-oriented couples therapy on depression: A randomized clinical trial. *Journal of Consulting and Clinical Psychology*, 76(6), 944–54.

Chasseguet-Smirgel, J. (1975). *The ego ideal.* New York: W. W. Norton.

Churchill, R., Moore, T. H., Furukawa, T. A., Caldwell, D. M., Davies, P., Jones, H., Shinohara, K., Imai, H., Lewis, G. & Hunot, V. (2013). 'Third wave' cognitive and behavioural therapies versus treatment as usual for depression. *Cochrane Database of Systematic Reviews*, 10th edn.

Cooper, A. & Lousada, J. (2005). *Borderline welfare: Feeling and fear of feeling in modern welfare.* London: Karnac Books.

Corrigan, F. M. & Hull, A. M. (2014). Neglect of the complex: Why psychotherapy for post-traumatic clinical presentations is often ineffective. *Psychiatric Bulletin*, 10, 1–4.

Cummins, A. M. (2002). 'The road to hell is paved with good intentions': Quality assurance as a social defence against anxiety. *Organisational and Social Dynamics: An International Journal of Psychoanalytic, Systemic and Group Relations Perspectives*, 2(1), 99–119.

Department of Health (2010). *Realizing the benefits: IAPT at full roll-out.* London: Department of Health.

Department of Health (DoH) (2011). *Which talking therapy for depression?* London: Department of Health.

Draper, D. (2006). The virtues of therapy. *Guardian*, 31 October.

Feltham, C. & Horton, I. (eds) (2012). *The Sage handbook of counselling and psychotherapy.* London: Sage.

Foucault, M. (1984a). On the genealogy of ethics: An overview of work in progress. *The Foucault Reader*, 340–72.

Foucault, M. (1984b). Truth and power. In P. Rabinow (ed.), *The Foucault Reader* (pp. 51–75). New York: Pantheon.

Foucault, M., Martin, L. H., Gutman, H. & Hutton, P. H. (1988). *Technologies of the self: A seminar with Michel Foucault.* Amherst, MA: University of Massachusetts Press.

Frankl, V. E. (1985). *Man's search for meaning.* New York: Simon and Schuster.

Freud, S. (1958). Observations on transference-love (further recommendations on the technique of psycho-analysis III). *Standard Edition*, 12, 157–71. London: Hogarth Press, 1923, 1–59.

Griffiths, S. & Steen, S. (2013). Improving Access to Psychological Therapies (IAPT) programme: Setting key performance indicators in a more robust context: A new perspective. *The Journal of Psychological Therapies in Primary Care*, 2(2), 133–41.

Griffiths, S., Foster, J., Steen, S. & Pietroni, P. (2013). *Mental health's market experiment: Commissioning psychological therapies through Any Qualified Provider.* Chester, PA: University of Chester Press.

Harvey, A., Watkins, E., Mansell, W. & Shafran, R. (2004). *Cognitive behavioural processes across psychological disorders: A transdiagnostic approach to research and treatment.* Oxford: Open University Press.

Help to Get and Stay in Work (2014). *Let's Talk.* Retrieved 2 January 2015 from www.lets-talk.co/what-kind-of-help-can-i-get/help-to-get-and-stay-in-work/.

Hoggett, P. (2010). Perverse social structures. *Journal of Psycho-Social Studies*, 4(1), 1–8.

Hood, C. (1991). A public management for all seasons? *Public Administration*, 69(1), 3–19.

House, R. & Loewenthal, D. (eds) (2008). *Against and for CBT: Towards a constructive dialogue?* Ross-on-Wye, UK: PCCS Books.

IAPT (2011). *Psychological wellbeing practitioners: Best practice guidelines.* London.

Langs, R. J. (1979). Truth therapy/lie therapy. *International Journal of Psychoanalytic Psychotherapy*, 8, 3–34.

Lasch, C. (1979). *The culture of narcissism: American life in an age of diminishing expectations.* New York: Norton.

Layard, R., Bell, S., Clark, D. M., Knapp, M., Meacher, M. & Priebe, S. (2006). *The depression report: A new deal for depression and anxiety disorders.* London: The centre for economic performance's mental health policy group, London School of Economics.

Leader, D. (2008). A quick fix for the soul? *Guardian*, 9 September 2008.

Lemma, A., Target, M. & Fonagy, P. (2011). *Brief dynamic interpersonal therapy: A clinician's guide.* Oxford: Oxford University Press.

McInnes, B. (2014). The researcher: And so, again, to IAPT. *Therapy Today*, 25(10), 18–24.

Menzies-Lyth, I. (1959). The functioning of social systems as a defence against anxiety. *Human Relations*, 13, 95–121.

Morrison, A. P. & Barratt, S. (2010). What are the components of CBT for psychosis? A Delphi study. *Schizophrenia Bulletin*, 36(1), 136–42.

Norcross, J. C. & Lambert, M. J. (2011). Evidence-based therapy relationships: Psychotherapy relationships that work, *Evidence-Based Responsiveness*, 2, 3–23.

Norcross, J. C. & Wampold, B. E. (2011). Evidence-based therapy relationships: Research conclusions and clinical practices. In J. C. Norcross (ed.), *Psychotherapy relationships that work: Evidence-based responsiveness* (2nd edn, pp. 423–30). New York: Oxford University Press.

Power, M. (1997a). *The audit society: Rituals of verification.* Oxford: Oxford University Press.

Reynolds, L. & McKee, M. (2012). 'Any qualified provider' in NHS reforms: But who will qualify? *The Lancet*, 379(9821), 1083–1084.

Rimke, H. & Brock, D. (2011). The culture of therapy: Psychocentrism in everyday life. In D. Brock, T. Thomas & R. Raby (eds), *Power and everyday practices* (pp. 183–203). New York: Springer.

Rizq, R. (2012). The perversion of care: Psychological therapies in a time of IAPT. *Psychodynamic Practice*, 18(1), 7–24.

Rogers, E. S., Chamberlin, J., Ellison, M. L. & Crean, T. (1997). A consumer-constructed scale to measure empowerment among users of mental health services. *Psychiatric Services*, 48(8), 1042–1047.

Rose, N. (1990). *Governing the soul: The shaping of the private self.* London: Taylor & Francis/Routledge.

Samuels, A. & Veale, D. (2009). Improving access to psychological therapies: For and against. *Psychodynamic Practice*, 15(1), 41–56.

Scanlon, C. & Adlam, J. (2010). The recovery model or the modelling of a cover-up? On the creeping privatisation and individualisation of dis-ease and being-unwell-ness. *Groupwork*, 20(3), 100–14.

Schmidt, N. B. & Woolaway-Bickel, K. (2000). The effects of treatment compliance on outcome in cognitive-behavioral therapy for panic disorder: Quality versus quantity. *Journal of Consulting and Clinical Psychology*, 68(1), 13–18.

Slade, M. & Priebe, S. (2001). Are randomised controlled trials the only gold that glitters? *The British Journal of Psychiatry*, 179(4), 286–87.

Terkel, S. (1978). Danger as a career. *Social Problems: Institutional and Interpersonal Perspectives*, 51, 51–5.

World Health Organization (2001). *Social determinants of mental health*. Geneva, Switzerland: WHO.

World Health Organization (2014). *Mental health atlas*. Retrieved 3 July 2014 from www.who.int/mental_health/evidence/atlas/mental_health_atlas_2014/.

8

WORKING IN PARTNERSHIP WITH IAPT

John Nuttall

Many have questioned the motives and underlying values that determined the introduction of the Improving Access to Psychological Therapies (IAPT) scheme in 2007. The fact that its chief architects were either economists or psychiatrists suggests that economic and scientific values prevailed, although certainly an intended outcome of the scheme was also an improvement in social well-being (Layard, 2006). Nevertheless, a key objective was to reduce unemployment and social incapacity benefit payments and, at least in the initial stages, one of its measures was the number of unemployed returning to work. It seems, nowadays, that monetary and economic value is the common metric we place on almost everything and by which, in the West at least, we seek to measure success and our lives. Economic laws, which inevitably control our lives, even lead us to reduce the analysis of health and well-being to a monetary base so that comparative judgements can be made about illnesses and resource allocation (UKCP, 2014). Oscar Wilde described a cynic as 'one who knows the price of everything and the value of nothing' and this adage raises the issue about how we value artefacts, social or other, and the different sets of values that exist in our current world. Gordon Allport (1961), one of the founding fathers of the humanistic psychology movement, distinguished six categories of life values – economic, political, scientific, social, aesthetic and spiritual. He made no judgement as to whether one set had or should have more importance than another. These categories, if universal, probably have different roles or emphases in different contexts, for example, across cultural and historical divides. Currently, we seem to place economic and scientific values ahead of those concerning the social, the aesthetic or the spiritual. With regard to the issue being considered in this book we might substitute the descriptors 'psychological' for aesthetic or spiritual and 'medical' for scientific, but clearly a conflict of values is evident in the debates currently raging in the health provision sector.

Notwithstanding this and the interference of economic recession, a welcome consequence of the IAPT scheme has been an increase of about £400 million into the woefully inadequate provision for the treatment of mental ill-health (LSE, 2012). This was further supported in 2012 when the Coalition Government introduced the Health and Social Care Act promising parity of esteem, if not immediately of resources, for mental and physical illness. However, the arrival of IAPT was greeted with some scepticism, dismay and protest by the counselling and psychological therapy professions. Its published ambition, to improve provision of psychological therapies in primary care, was heralded, on the one hand, as necessary and laudable, and yet, on the other hand, as a potential danger to the rich and varied supply of therapeutic services and approaches that had evolved to meet the needs of local communities. The requirement, initially determined by NICE guidelines, to provide therapies that met the criteria of evidence-based practice (EBP) meant the main therapeutic approach proposed would be cognitive behavioural therapy (CBT). This was based on clinical research studies that indicate this as the most effective intervention for what seem to be the dominant presenting problems in primary care of depression and anxiety. CBT's apparently systematised delivery and predictable outcomes made the economic objectives of reduced unemployment and social benefit payments seem attainable (Layard, 2006).

The pervading dialectic

Given that substantial community-based resources were already in place, there was considerable controversy about the necessity and value of introducing such a highly structured scheme, and concern that economic motives were leading politicians to look for solutions in the easiest rather than the best place (Loewenthal & House, 2010). Mulla Nasrudin warned us of such tendencies centuries ago (Shah, 1971):

> On one occasion a friend found him on his knees in the street looking for something.
> 'What have you lost Mulla?' he asked.
> 'My key' replied Nasrudin.
> After a few minutes of helping him search, the neighbour asked, 'where did you drop it?'
> 'At home', said the Mulla.
> 'Then why, for heaven's sake are we looking here?'
> 'Well, there's more light here' replied Nasrudin.

Is it easier to seek answers 'in the street' of economic and scientific values, though they might be better sought 'at home' in social, aesthetic or spiritual values? Clearly there is a need to improve mental illness provision, and equally a need to do this cost effectively (LSE, 2012). The economic, political and scientific/medical values that underpin the imperative of such a cost–benefit scheme would inevitably come into dialectic relationship with the social, psychological/aesthetic and spiritual values that traditionally pervade the provision of such community-based services. This dialectic is no better emphasised than in a motto from Ambroise Pare (1510–1590) quoted by Freud, 'Je le pansai, Dieu le guerit' ['I dressed the wound, God healed him'] (Roazen, 1974, p. 185). Recently, it has been illustrated in a report by Altson et al. (2014) of therapists working in current IAPT settings, which identified tension between two discourses. One constructs IAPT as a powerful bureaucratic medical 'black box' (Altson, 2014) in which therapists lose their identity, while the other constructs therapists as maintaining a personal view of themselves, outside the scheme, as caring, self-determining and well-trained individuals. These tensions are noticeable even in commercially based institutions serving the community, such as banks. In their chase for economic values of wealth creation and reward, they abandoned traditional banking values centred around thrift, temperance and community. This seems, at least superficially, to have been restored recently in advertising slogans such as 'Goodbye unfair banking – Hello Natwest' and 'Halifax – always giving you extra'. How deep-rooted and meaningful this dialectic about values is to the psychotherapy professions was brought into focus by Jung, 'but were it not a fact of experience that supreme values reside in the soul, psychology would not interest me in the least, for the soul would then be nothing but a miserable vapour' (Jung, 1944, par. 14).

The impact at community level

For over ten years I have been the Chair of Trustees and one of several honorary psychotherapists of a charity in West London that contributed to the rich and varied supply of therapeutic services referred to above. In the context of the issues discussed in this book, I should like to describe how the advent and operations of IAPT were experienced and managed by this charity. The future course of such provision seems now open for debate and should be of concern to all stakeholders interested in the effective delivery of psychological services in primary care.

West London Community Counselling (WLCC) began in the 1980s as a small bereavement agency. By the millennium it had grown into a service supplying 'free' counselling to the local community attracting funds from local social services and the regional NHS Trust. Referrals came primarily from local GPs and associated medical services such as community mental health teams and hospitals. The charity at this time depended on funding from a narrow range of state sources with corresponding contractual conditions. It had become, like many charities in the sector, a supplier to the local health service taking unwitting advantage of volunteer trainees; albeit organised by a few professionals for the purpose. The *quid pro quo* of such an arrangement is the opportunity it provides for trainees and newly qualified practitioners to gain experience with clients, a basic requirement of all professional training. Such arrangements, up and down the country, hide the true cost of providing psychological services that would otherwise require much greater resource by having to employ adequately paid professionals. As a system of provision it is ethically controversial in that it encourages people into a poorly resourced profession where volunteer trainees occupy the very jobs they hope to be remunerated for when they qualify.

WLCC initially occupied a small number of rooms rented in a local office block but as it grew it moved to larger leased premises in Shepherd's Bush. However, shortly after the move there was an unpredicted tightening of local government and NHS funding which was cut by a third in one year. A number of staff had to be made redundant and others worked part-time until funding was replaced over the next few years from the National Lottery and other third-sector sources. Eventually, state sector funds were reinstated as the new Primary Care Trust (PCT) established itself. During this time, the charity was renamed West London Centre for Counselling and a new management and Board of Trustees were in place. They resolved to boost the charity's reserves and diversify its source of funds, and introduced a number of key performance indicators concerning cost per counselling hour, outcome evaluation and financial rigour. CORE was introduced as the primary outcome measure, and a panel of independent clinical advisers was appointed to moderate procedures and operational dilemmas. At this point, non-state funding was raised to around 40 per cent of total income and these measures ushered in a period of stability and steady growth. Annual receptions were held at prestigious local venues, including the BBC and Houses of Parliament, for all stakeholders to receive an update on the agency's progress. This improvement raised the confidence of the local PCT commissioners, GPs and care services, and money began to flow with more certainty and consistency from these sources.

It is a paradox that such success brings its own problems and dilemmas. As funds grew from state sources and financial reserves were built to withstand future shocks, smaller and more diverse sources of funds seemed more difficult to attract. Charitable sources of funds such as those associated with banks, livery companies, industry and even the National Lottery seemed reluctant to support the operations of what they perceived to be successful and well-resourced operation. Heraclitus pointed out, 'the path up and down the mountain is one and the same', and this paradox is an example of what the alchemists called the *coincidentia oppositorum* – the coincidence of opposites. So, what provides advantage might have within it unintended or hidden disadvantages. This made WLCC less stable and less autonomous as funds, once again, became concentrated from the sources with which it was contracted. Charities in this position become more like business partners and suppliers of front-line services, with potentially less autonomy to do the kind of work they wish to do and can best undertake and provide. Nevertheless, WLCC continued to attract a small level of funds from diverse sources which supported the development of new projects such as group therapy and couples counselling and helped with asset and infra-structure renewal. By around 2008, WLCC employed a team of five qualified staff and engaged about 80 volunteer counsellors and supervisors to deal with approximately 1,700 referrals and deliver some 8,000 hours of counselling per annum. It offered a mix of therapeutic approaches, albeit in the form of a 12-session model, extendable in certain situations. Relationship with all its stakeholders was open, transparent and solid. However, another cloud began to form over this relatively stable and sunny scenario.

The advent of Improving Access to Psychological Therapies

Before IAPT, individuals in need of psychological therapy could seek help from a range of services either by self-referral, or via a variety of services. A person seeking help through their GP might have found themselves referred for counselling to a range of resources that included independent counsellors, local and national charities (such as WLCC, MIND), specialist agencies (for HIV, drug and alcohol, domestic violence etc.) and psychological services in hospitals and community mental health centres. Also, there was often referral between and across such services until the most appropriate intervention was determined. Although rich in referral options and therapeutic approaches, this provision was, overall, poorly organised, badly measured and grossly under-funded. It relied, as mentioned above, substantially on charitable services using trainees and newly qualified professionals.

WLCC was one of such services in West London and in a study of local provision stood out as one of the most efficient and cost effective service providers in the area. WLCC had introduced CORE alongside its own user satisfaction survey, with outcomes that matched national norms. Its cost of delivery was at the lower end of a range that stretched from £40 to £200 per counselling hour. Notwithstanding such pockets of excellence, IAPT aimed to bring coherence to primary care provision by introducing a highly structured system of referral, assessment, treatment and outcome measurement that would achieve specific targets in terms of community access and employment prospects for those with psychological distress.

In some communities the introduction of IAPT led to a significant sweeping aside of the above ad-hoc provisions while in other areas 'partnerships' with existing providers were encouraged, especially if these were well managed charities. The fear within the therapy professions as this policy proceeded was that it would impose a particular model of therapy and jeopardise the employment and training prospects of therapists and trainees providing the wide range of therapies available. There was also the survival fear that if the 'partners' did not conform to the IAPT system either in its operations or its model of therapy, NHS funding would be withdrawn, the system imposed and NHS referrals that would otherwise sustain the partner be diverted. It is unlikely within this scenario that local charitable agencies could survive, putting in jeopardy both client choice and training facilities for would-be counsellors and therapists. IAPT adheres to guidelines set by the National Institute for Clinical Excellence (NICE), directing which psychological therapies should be provided at primary care level. In the early stages these guidelines recommended CBT as the most effective treatment. However, by 2011 a developing agenda calling for more patient choice emerged and the newly formed Clinical Commissioning Groups, which succeeded PCTs, are now challenged to commission provision of an additional four therapy interventions recognised by NICE (IAPT, 2012). These are Counselling for Depression, Interpersonal Therapy, Dynamic Interpersonal Therapy and Couples Therapy for Depression. Although there is some deference to non-CBT approaches in this, the manualised nature of their delivery still pays homage to the psychiatric-medical dogma of condition-diagnosis-treatment-predictable outcome. Indeed these interventions, which suddenly appear manualised and evidence-based, pose an affront to the four-year post-graduate training typically undertaken by UKCP accredited psychotherapists.

Coincidentia oppositorum

The danger as the policy developed was that, contrary to the good intentions of the scheme, it was and is in danger of resulting in its opposite. As Paul Burstow, MP and Minister of State for Care Services, stated in 2010, 'At the moment IAPT is a little too much like Henry Ford's business philosophy . . . you can have any therapy as long as it's CBT' (BACP, 2014, p. 4). If I might add to the analogy there was also the danger of only being able to obtain it from one dealer, wherever that might be. Client choice of therapy in terms of both modality and convenience of access (location) was seriously threatened as IAPT treatment centres concentrated resources and narrowed the diagnostic criteria eligible for treatment (ibid.).

The above paradox and consequent anxieties were constantly debated and present within the management and trustee meetings of WLCC in the advent period. Questions about the continuity of funding, the status of the agency within the community, and recognition of the quality of work dominated as the introduction of the IAPT scheme grew closer. Alongside this came the re-organisation of local primary care services as a new Clinical Commissioning Group (CCG) succeeded the old Primary Care Trust. Local commissioners seemed unsure of their new responsibilities and, for what seemed months on end, were unable to determine or confirm the continuity of funding for WLCC or its status alongside the proposed IAPT scheme, which was called promisingly *Back-on-track*. The trustees drew up outline contingency plans for survival or closure in case funding and referrals were substantially cut. There was a feeling of disbelief and some level of denial of what might happen. It seemed inconceivable to dismantle such an efficient and effective resource to replace it with a single 'one size fits all' provision at what, in their estimation, would be considerably higher cost to the community. Indeed there was some consternation in the early days when it was rumoured that the rent IAPT were paying for their offices was alone equal to the entire annual running costs of WLCC.

Among the trustees, the clash of values inherent in the charity's activities was brought into focus. The social, spiritual and aesthetic values at the heart of this kind of charity were being compromised or attacked by the economic and political values filtering down from government institutions and politicians ostensibly of good virtue and intention. However, as Bertrand Russell (1935) argued in one of his Sceptical Essays called *The Harm That Good Men Do*, virtue does not always have desirable consequences. He satirically defined a good man as 'one whose opinions and activities are pleasing to the holders of power' (p. 87). And the holders of power seemed hell bent on cost effectiveness, measurement and predictability. So much so that some argue that the obsession with these aspects of the scheme represent a 'perversion of care ... used to mask the unbearable feelings of helplessness in the face of our limitations when trying to help those in psychological distress' (Rizq, 2012, p. 7). The psychic defence here is that the people in power feel they are 'doing' something against a rising tide of increasing incapacity caused by psychological stress. Rizq's views suggest that the unconscious processes at work, although conceived as benign, often manifest as malign. A similarly ominous perspective is supplied by Jung, who pointed out that our rational abilities are not always able to override our instinctual nature; what he called the 'Shadow', a dominant archetype of the collective unconscious. He pointed out,

> there is an unconscious psychic reality which demonstrably influences consciousness and its contents ... We still go on thinking and acting as before, as if we are *simplex* and not *duplex*. Accordingly, we imagine ourselves to be innocuous, reasonable and humane. It needs only an almost imperceptible disturbance of equilibrium in a few of our rulers' heads to plunge the world into blood, fire and radioactivity.
>
> *(Jung 1957, par. 561)*

Although Jung was alluding to the dangers of the Cold War he was nevertheless highlighting the capacity we have of being influenced by unconscious processes of a darker and perhaps more destructive or punitive nature. The idea that introducing a kind of factory system of psychological intervention that returns people to work, without any thought as to whether this exacerbates the nature of their problem, feels destructive and punitive. Sennett (2007) highlights the issue, 'The fragmentation of big institutions has left many people's lives in a fragmented state: the places they work more resembling train stations than villages as family life is disoriented by the demands of work' (p. 2). He posits the need for a whole new attitude where individuals have to learn to manage short-term and fragmented relationships, develop and change their skills base, and let go of any ideas that past experience and skills provide future prospects. I wonder if the Shadow of the IAPT system, although a defence against anxiety, is identification with an aggressor that demands compliance and disciplined rehabilitation so that people become the hard working tax payers the economy requires.

Sennett's new attitude implies, at least, an adaptation of the familiar protestant work ethic (Weber, 1930) which is characterised by the growth of large bureaucratic institutions (banks, companies, public sector) in which we all must play our contributory role. IAPT is yet another 'institution', in this sense, helping those unable to 'do' to become 'doers' again. This highlights another aspect of our dual nature identified by the psychologist, Erich Fromm. In his book, *To Have or To Be* (Fromm, 1976), he argued that there are two basic and opposed modes of existence. One is aimed at having and owning, and the other at being and living. This aspect of our nature has also been recognised in various traditions and is perhaps manifest in the effect economic values, aims and constraints have on our daily lives and the environment. It is one interpretation of the Fall of Adam in that his temptation to have (knowledge) forfeited his right to 'be' anxiety free, and he was cast out 'to do' for himself. In recompense, most of the world's religions espouse values associated with abstinence of material possessions and desires and the redemption offered by hard work and good deeds. Fromm (1976) believed and wrote that 'For the first time in history the physical survival of the human race depends on a radical change of the human heart' (p. 19). Following the latest economic crisis and the parallel rise in incapacity due to mental ill-health there is a conceptual question as to whether the protestant work ethic influencing the IAPT scheme requires such a 'change of the human heart'.

Working towards shared values

Notwithstanding such views, in 2009 the local CCG, cognisant of WLCC's excellent work and reputation, proposed a new contract for provision of services on the understanding that the Centre worked in partnership with the new IAPT service. A substantial increase in funds was indicated, but also a substantially different way of working and monitoring would be required. At a trustees' meeting in 2010 a rigorous, if subdued, debate took place about the effects of such a partnership. There was some irritation that there was not much option to refuse the proposal, and there was also concern about the clash of values it implied. Were the economic and scientific values of cost effectiveness and treatment measurement overriding those of the social and psychological values of choice, diversity and care? Such questions prompted WLCC's trustees to write specifically to the CCG commissioners asserting their right and responsibility to manage the charity as they saw fit in accordance with its articles of association. At the same board meeting a decision was made to cooperate and introduce the necessary changes to WLCC's general model of provision. The local commissioners responded both constructively and positively acknowledging WLCC's independence and allaying fears of losing autonomy. Following some further negotiation the following operational parameters were agreed upon:

- Direct referrals from GPs would cease and be channelled through the IAPT (*Back-on-track*) triage team;
- the outcome measures of GAD7 and PHQ9 would be introduced;
- WLCC would provide on-site facilities for three IAPT personnel to provide CBT sessions;
- at some later date, additional salaried counsellors should be employed to add to the agency's professional expertise;
- access to the centralised computer system (IAPTus) for the collection of client data, including all the weekly outcome scores, was to be arranged;
- WLCC would accept an appropriate share of the overall target of providing therapeutic intervention to 15 per cent of the local population with psychological difficulties per annum.

However, three important aspects were retained that represented the fundamental values that WLCC felt it embodied:

*   the current twelve session model could remain;
*   the overall counselling approach was recognised as NICE compliant, of high quality and in line with BACP requirements;
*   the use of advanced trainee volunteers could be maintained.

In addition, WLCC would be free to raise its own funds to extend its services into other therapeutic modalities and diagnostic categories as it wished, although it would not be able to offer these services to patients referred via *Back-on-track*. These arrangements were somewhat of a relief and offered some hope that the IAPT managers and local commissioners were recognising the benefit of choice and the variety of therapeutic approaches offered. *Back-on-track* itself would provide the triage, CBT and other NICE specified therapies through the recruitment and training of its own personnel. WLCC would be an adjunct to this provision, dealing only with the specific diagnostic categories of depression and anxiety, and be remunerated according to the client numbers seen. So, contrary to perceived fears and ad hoc accounts from other localities the scheme provided substantial additional funding for existing provision while imposing compliance with a structure for referral and outcome measurement. The optimistic view from this is that IAPT need not be the all or nothing provision feared. WLCC's historical close ties with local GPs and commissioners enabled the arguments for client choice and the efficacy of a range of approaches to be heard. This was to the benefit and not the demise of the existing provision, and gives hope for a future moulding of the scheme to expand patient choice and expertise of provision without losing the economic goals that allow increased funding.

The negotiating process, with the allied anxiety of annihilation, was nevertheless experienced as mildly oppressive, with a new discourse around provision dominating thinking and operational priorities. Despite a relatively positive outcome, WLCC lost its identity as a local charity doing good works and overnight became a subcontractor to the most powerful service provider in the sector. There was a sense in which WLCC had survived, but at some cost to its autonomy, its caring ethos, and perhaps its future as a provider of placements for trainee counsellors. The question remains whether such a powerful force that draws on significantly different values, such as economic and scientific, can work alongside and effectively harness resources that have a different value base. This dissonance is evident in a report published in 2012 by the London School of Economics and Political Science, *How Mental Illness Loses Out in the NHS* (LSE, 2012). While vehemently arguing the need for increased funding for mental ill-health provision based on Quality-adjusted life-years analysis, the report's recommendations point out,

> IAPT is already preparing itself for a commissioning system where services are paid according to the outcomes of their patients. This is a welcome

development. And so is the practice of competitive tender which is already well-established in IAPT. But IAPT insists that the treatments provided are evidence-based and recommended by NICE. This is exactly the same as the practice in physical medicine, and we would strongly oppose any system where providers could be paid for providing treatments without a strong evidential base.

(p. 18)

This is another report from a group headed by Professor Lord Richard Layard, composed almost entirely of members with titles that suggest, at least, a heavy orientation towards economic, political and scientific values. Their strategic aims might be considered virtuous and in line with those of the therapy professions, but it remains to be seen if in meeting them operationally these values can be realistically synthesised with those espoused by the people tasked to deliver.

Working together

This difference in values was not ultimately manifest or detrimental to the provision in practice, owing substantially to the view of the local commissioners recognising the high quality of service provided by WLCC and their willingness to acknowledge its independent status. However, in a number of operational areas the different underlying values are apparent and the effects of the partnership can be discussed broadly under the themes taken from the BACP document *Psychological Therapies and Parity of Esteem* (2014).

Access: Provision in the community has substantially improved in that the scheme is delivering on its targets of attending to 15 per cent of the estimated population needing psychological intervention. This is commendable, and local targets have increased in view of this as the local scheme is being held up as an exemplary model. Nevertheless the difference in values is present below the surface as 'attending to' is defined as patients meeting the criteria of two clinical contacts – one of which is always the telephone triage and the second might be only a letter of appointment. Neither of these in psychotherapy practice would be considered clinical contact of any benefit. Physical access is now concentrated into three locations within the scheme area and although this seems adequate in view of the available transport facilities the closure in the area of several specialist charities has, arguably, reduced the choice of help available.

Waiting times: Prior to IAPT, patients were referred directly from GPs and waiting times for assessment and treatment were within two to three weeks. GPs now refer to a triage team following which there is further referral for treatment. In the early period of the scheme waiting times for treatment sometimes extended to several weeks. However, the effect of this was interesting and two-fold. First, the added complexity and waiting time for access seemed to have a paradoxical effect on patients' subsequent attendance. Average session attendance at WLCC increased from five to eight sessions of the 12 offered. Second, *Back-on-track* initiated a 'fast-track' triage process by which GP referrals for counselling could be passed immediately to WLCC. Overall, the scheme now meets targeted waiting times, comparable to the pre-IAPT period for WLCC, and session attendance has improved.

Choice: Government stated policy has been to extend patient choice in the NHS, although this has so far been primarily implemented in secondary care. As discussed earlier there is anxiety in the professions about restricting the choice of therapies available through IAPT and the threat this poses to training programmes and the rich diversity available. The partnership approach has allowed pluralism (Cooper & McLeod, 2007) and variety to continue, albeit within a narrow diagnostic range of mild to medium depression or anxiety as identified by the *Back-on-track* triage procedure. WLCC now sees approximately one third of the referrals in the area, which still amount to around 1,500 clients annually. Other diagnostic categories are referred elsewhere for different treatments regimes the most prominent of which is CBT and its allied approaches. As part of the partnership arrangement and to offer patients the choice of location WLCC provides consulting rooms and computer stations for three CBT practitioners directly employed by *Back-on-track*.

Services and staffing: Within the debate that healthcare clinicians should have an understanding of mental and physical health and their interrelationship, it is asserted that those working in the arena of mental health need a sound training in psychological therapies and assessment. The majority of the new IAPT workforce are Psychological Wellbeing Practitioners (PWPs) who have limited experience of face to face therapeutic practice and assessment (IAPT, 2011). They undertake the triage via telephone with the aid of computer based questionnaires and diagnostics. WLCC feels it prudent to undertake an additional assessment of clients referred, using its own professionally trained assessors, and in a significant percentage of cases decline referrals as clinically inappropriate. Charities, like WLCC, employ professional therapists and engage advanced trainees, usually on masters and doctoral level courses accredited by the BACP, UKCP or BPS. This is a well-trained resource capable of providing expert and cost effective intervention; a capability acknow-ledged by the local commissioners in this case. However, in many regions this expertise, with its integrative and pluralistic nature, is finding it difficult to meet the precepts of EBP and the manualised treatment regime this requires. And yet evidence is growing that this kind of provision is showing significantly good outcome results on the measures (PHQ9, GAD7) introduced. Overall outcome measures are meeting expectations although *Back-on-track* seems unable to isolate WLCC specific results. Consequently, and as a defence against the fears discussed, the Centre has re-instated CORE as an additional internal measure. This continues to show the efficacy of such a pluralistic provision in that outcomes match those expected and established by CORE nationally. With some deference to this, the CCG met their commitment to fund the employment of additional counsellors as referrals grew.

Funding: the partnership brought significantly more funding to WLCC, but with the consequence of a loss of autonomy and anxiety around compliance and future dependency. Such a relationship evokes the tension between fears of engulfment and abandonment, redolent of the core complex (Glasser, 1997), we have to deal with in our patients. There is a struggle, in complying with the day-to-day bureaucracy, not to lose focus on the social and psychological values that underpin the history and ethos of the charitable project. Trustee board meetings easily become dominated by monitoring and measurement instead of the social benefit of the work being undertaken. This is not ameliorated by attendance on IAPT committees which are equally obsessed with numerical targets and policies from 'on high', without much consideration of their social effect, clinical efficacy or partnership implications. The danger is that, as more money is provided, the increased need for accountability and evidence will eat away at the values at the core of psychological therapists, whose work identity lies in the social consequences of their endeavours. If this happens patients are in danger of internalising this attitude with the possible result of worsening rather than improving the nation's mental health (Sennett, 2007).

This relatively optimistic scenario of co-operation and synthesis at the operational level, however, hides the lack of power experienced at the strategic level (Altson, 2014). Although managers of WLCC are invited to the local IAPT board meetings they have little say in the implementation of the strategic directives handed down. The NHS and IAPT are perhaps the last vestiges of Weberian bureaucracy (Weber, 1930) in the current neo-liberal age. 'Weber is almost exclusively concerned with what the bureaucratic structure attains: precision, reliability, efficiency', asserts Merton (1970, p. 85), who goes on to ask, 'What are the limitations of the organisation designed to attain these goals?' (ibid.). He elaborates:

> The chief merit of bureaucracy is its technical efficiency, with a premium placed on precision, speed, expert control, continuity, discretion and optimal returns on output. The structure is one which approaches the complete elimination of personalised relationships and non-rational considerations (hostility, anxiety, affectual involvement etc).
>
> *(Merton, 1970, p. 84)*

It is hard to imagine a system less appropriate for the provision of recovery from psychological distress. Notwithstanding this, WLCC has kept its identity and autonomy and continues with activities close to its own work ethic. Small levels of ad hoc funds have been forthcoming from third-sector donors and loyal followers of its work that have allowed expansion into group therapy and relationship counselling. And in order to meet future obligations to the IAPT scheme, the agency plans to incorporate training in the new approaches being recommended by NICE.

Conclusion

Within any financially constrained community service, whether a state or private enterprise, there is a tension between the values associated with having to supply it cost effectively and the ideals of the service itself. Cost effectiveness implies measurement, monitoring, targets and reward, whereas the ideals of service involve compassion, relationship, holism and pluralism. Merton (1970) points out the ambivalence and ambiguity inherent in any bureaucratic system that attempts this. In this chapter I have attempted to elucidate this ambivalence as it applies to the IAPT scheme and the conflict of values this represents. This does not mean that one set of values is necessarily more virtuous than another, only that there is a tension that needs resolution. WLCC's understanding and negotiation of this tension has proved fruitful for the implementation and running of the scheme in its area. WLCC has managed a synthesis of different values sets, partly through negotiation and a sense of self-worth, and partly through deference and understanding of what needs to be achieved in an era of limited resource.

No doubt in negotiating the ambivalence the trustees and managers of the charity drew on their knowledge base in psychotherapy and the need to achieve balance between what is a given and what can be self-determined. This involves balancing the internal conflict between the fears of engulfment and isolation and avoiding regression to basic assumption functioning (Bion, 1970). There is always the tendency to resort to the basic assumption of dependency with the belief that some higher force, such as a professional body, or the local MP, or people of influence you know, will resolve the issues. Indeed I believe the profession itself has to be careful of the subtle nature of this unconscious tendency whose aim is to dissipate anxiety to the point of inaction or explosion (ibid., p. 125). Synthesising such diverse values requires a particular attitude, which Russell (1961) espoused when studying a philosopher, but which I think is applicable in this case:

> the right attitude is neither reverence nor contempt, but first a kind of hypothetical sympathy, until it is possible to know what it feels like to believe in his theories, and only then a revival of the critical attitude, which should resemble, as far as possible, the state of mind of a person abandoning opinions which he has hitherto held. Contempt interferes with the first part of this process, and reverence with the second.
>
> (p. 58)

The Roman stoic Seneca argued that wisdom was the most perfect of the virtues and believed, in the long run, the perfectly wise person would act in harmony with all the virtues. I believe there is a set of qualities *sine qua non* within us that might lead to a beneficent synthesis of values. The first is individuation, the development of self-awareness, self-acceptance and autonomy. It involves gaining awareness of disagreeable aspects of the self and accepting them for what they are – thoughts and feelings that may be unwanted and are in the broad sense aspects of our Shadow. Thus we can avoid the derived behaviours which ultimately determine how we relate to others. The second is aspiration. This enables self-direction and gives us the capacity to choose our behaviours, goals and desires. This may be an organismic faculty in us all, which provides motivation, drive and curiosity. Existentially, it situates us on the cusp of the future, at a point where we can decide not to be determined by the past or present but be drawn forward by our potential. The next is solicitude. Some consider this a fundamental condition of a human Being (Heidegger, 1962; Scheler, 1970). For me this involves love and care for ourselves and others. It brings the willingness and ability to acknowledge and understand, if not always accept, the Shadow in others. This allows us enjoyment in life and to engage and relate to others; to have empathy for, and understand the values of, others without losing autonomy or the aspiration to be who we want to be. The fourth concerns congruence – one of the core conditions of humanistic counselling. This involves feeling 'joined up' and connected and brings the ability to be tolerant, hold ambivalence and paradox and remain optimistic in the face of disappointment when our goals and values are challenged. This may involve adapting our values, objectives and relationships while maintaining autonomy, purpose, and caring. These are the qualities all parties need to engage in when considering and determining what could be the most significant change in governmental and public attitudes and financial resources, with regard to mental illness provision in decades.

References

Allport, G. (1961). *Patterns and growth in personality*. New York: Holt, Rinehart & Winston.

Altson, C. (2014). What are the perceived implications, if any, for non-IAPT therapists working in an IAPT service? Presentation at the *University Psychotherapy and Counselling Association Conference*, November 2014.

Altson, C., Loewenthal, D., Gaitanidis, A. & Thomas, R. (2014). What are the perceived implications, if any, for non-IAPT therapists working in an IAPT service? *British Journal of Guidance and Counselling*. Published online 02 October 2014.

BACP (2014). *Psychological therapies and parity of esteem: From commitment to reality*. Lutterworth, UK: BACP.

Bion, W. R. (1970). *Experience in groups*. London: Routledge.

Cooper, M. & McLeod, J. (2007). A pluralistic framework for counselling and psychotherapy: Implications for research. *Counselling and Psychotherapy Research*, 7(3), 35–143.

Fromm, E. (1976). *To have or to be*. London: Abacus.

Glasser, M. (1997). Aggression and sadism in the perversions. In I. Rosen (ed.), *Sexual deviation* (3rd edn). Oxford: Oxford University Press.

Heidegger, M. (1962). *Being and time*. J. Macquarrie & E. Robinson (trans.). Oxford: Blackwell.

IAPT (2011). *Psychological wellbeing practitioners: Best practice guidelines*. London: NHS.

IAPT (2012). *Guidance for commissioning IAPT training 2012/13*. London: NHS.

Jung, C. G. (1944). *Psychology and alchemy. Collected Works 12*. London: Routledge.

Jung, C. G. (1957). *The undiscovered self. Collected Works 10*. London: Routledge.

Layard, R. (2006). *The depression report: A new deal for depression and anxiety disorders*. London: LSE.

Loewenthal, D. & House, R. (2010). *Critically engaging CBT.* Maidenhead, UK: Open University Books.

LSE. (2012). *How mental illness loses out in the NHS: A report by The Centre for Economic Performance's Mental Health Policy Group.* London: LSE.

Merton, R. K. (1970). Bureaucratic structure and personality. In W. P. Sexton (ed.), *Organization theories.* Columbus, OH: Charles E. Merrill.

Rizq, R. (2012). The perversion of care: Psychological therapies in a time of IAPT. *Psychodynamic Practice,* 18(1), 7–24.

Roazen, P. (1974). *Freud and his followers.* Harmondsworth, UK: Penguin.

Russell, B. (1961). *History of western philosophy* (2nd edn). London: Allen and Unwin.

Scheler, M. F. (1970). *The nature of sympathy.* P. Heath (trans.). New York: Archon Books.

Sennett, R. (2007). *The culture of the new capitalism.* Yale, NH: Yale University Press.

Shah, I. (1971). *The Sufis.* New York: Anchor Books.

UKCP (2014). *Valuing mental health: How a subjective wellbeing approach can show just how much it matters.* London: UKCP.

Weber, M. (1930). *The Protestant ethic and the spirit of capitalism.* T. Parsons & A. Giddens (trans.). London & Boston: Allen and Unwin.

PART III

Mainly practice

9

PSYCHOTHERAPY IN AN AGE OF MANAGED CARE[1]

John Lees

> Psychoanalysis starts from the position that there is no cure, but that we need different ways of living with ourselves and different descriptions of these so-called selves.
>
> *Adam Phillips, Interview with Maria Popova*

Introduction

The neo-liberal New Public Management (NPM) approach to healthcare, with evidence-based practice underpinning it, has begun to have a strong influence on the field of counselling and psychotherapy (therapy), in the form of the Improved Access to Psychological Therapies (IAPT) scheme. However, during the same period since the 1980s, there has also been the emergence of a different paradigm based on a significant and extensive, but marginalized, approach to research into the counselling and psychotherapy (therapy) practice and a flowering of creative research methods.

Both of these approaches to practice and research have tended to peel off in different directions with little dialogue between them. This creates an unbalanced profession in which one approach takes the dominant position and creates a professional climate in which there is little 'liberty of thought and discussion', to use the words of the nineteenth century liberal philosopher John Stuart Mill. As he said in his work *On Liberty* in 1859 a healthy society cultivates an awareness of the fallibility of opinions, creates space for different opinions, attempts to eliminate prejudice in regard to points of view that are different from one's own and tries to overcome dogma (Roberts, 2004, p. 71). Translated into the therapy profession there needs to be 'more than one research discourse' since the dominant paradigm is 'open to error as is any activity of human beings' (Lees, 2005, p. 31).

My aim in this chapter is to see how we can create a greater balance between these two paradigms within the profession. My thoughts about this thus have an action research element; namely, 'to influence or change some aspect of whatever is the focus of the research' (Robson, 2002, p. 215).

In this chapter I will look at the different views on healing in these two paradigms and will reflect on how, in an ideal world, they might engage in constructive dialogue with each other in order to further the culture, and enhance the vibrancy, of the therapy profession. To develop this view I will look, first of all, at the dominant paradigm in order to identify some of its key features. I will then look at the marginalized approach to therapy practice and how it differs from managed care. Then I will examine the new creative research methods (which incorporate psychotherapeutic principles) which I will call transformational research. This discussion will then serve as preparation for the latter part of the chapter in which I will look at how the marginalized approach to therapy practice and transformational research might further constructive dialogue in the therapy profession in an age of managed care.

The dominant paradigm

NPM and IAPT are no different from government welfare policies in general in that 'welfare from the point of view of the State is almost always interwoven with social control, anxiety about the possible uppity behaviour of ordinary people' (Humphries, 2015). As a consequence of this, rather than enabling clients to unfold their potential, transform themselves and live a more fulfilled life, these schemes prioritize the needs of the State. In particular, they further its economic and business agenda. IAPT was originally designed to address the problem that 'between 1995 and 2005 about half a million extra people registered for Incapacity Benefit (IB). . . . because of a mental illness, taking the total to about 1.1 million' (O'Brien, 2013). The report, which formed the basis for the scheme, argued that psychological therapy has the potential to reduce the cost of IB 'for those unable to work due to psychological distress' (Layard, 2006). By early 2015 it had become a central part of government mental health policy, particularly in regard to depression and anxiety: 'from April 2016, 75 percent of patients with depression or anxiety disorders needing access to psychological therapies are to be treated within six weeks of referral, and 95 percent in 18 weeks' (NHS, 2015).

IAPT is orientated towards enabling individuals to develop the capacity to return to work as soon as possible but does not take into account the increasingly stressful and uncertain working conditions of life today which contribute to the problems in the first place as described by Sennett (1998) and others. These working conditions pose ever greater stresses on the workforce and create anxieties, not least because of perpetuating a fragmentary lifestyle where jobs are no longer for life and are increasingly insecure. As Sennett says: 'How can a human being develop a narrative of identity and life history in a society composed of episodes and fragments?' (1998, p. 26).

We can look at IAPT from many points of view. In this discussion I will look at it from the point of view of three fundamental principles – a centralized management system which mirrors the authority and hierarchies of the State, a focus on 'recovering from' symptoms and, finally, as a result of this, becoming resilient citizens in order to participate in social and economic life, a notion which is now quite widespread in healthcare research (Fisher & Lees, 2015). It aims to further the economic agenda of becoming strong enough to withstand the conditions that we encounter in society today. It aims to make us more resilient so as to serve the needs of the market – to make us useful consumers and producers. If we are not able to do this we are of little use to society and, in fact, we become a burden on it due to our need for incapacity benefits and other forms of social support. It adopts the same principles as the 'treatments' of the psychiatrist, Lewis Yelland, in his work with shell-shocked soldiers in World War I when he used electric shocks and exhorted traumatized soldiers to be heroes and not cowards in the service of the State's war machine (Herman, 1992, p. 21).

In neo-liberalism all spheres of society are centred on economic considerations. But there is more to society than the economy. In the 1920s Steiner (1923/1977) argued that a healthy society has three separate but interlinked spheres corresponding to the French revolution slogan of Liberté, Égalité, Fraternité – a cultural and spiritual sphere of individual freedom (Liberté), a legal and political sphere of individual rights (Égalité) and a sphere of economic activity where ideally we work in harmony and cooperation with each other with an appreciation of each other's contribution (Fraternité). But, in neo-liberalism, the economic sphere permeates the other two spheres. It acquires a moral (even spiritual) authority to mould our future by taking over the cultural sphere of Liberté and restricting individual freedom. It also determines our individual rights by overwhelming the sphere of Égalité with the principles of economic value. Finally, the ideal of Fraternité in economic life is replaced by a moral imperative to engage in competition which promotes the 'survival of the fittest'.

Developments in clinical practice

As managed care has developed since the 1980s there have been a number of parallel developments in therapy theory and practice which, if fully recognized and respected, have the potential to establish a balanced profession, for instance, the 'relational turn' in therapy which Aron (2014) dates from the publication of *Object Relations in Psychoanalytic Theory* by Greenberg and Mitchell in 1983. The frame of reference for this perspective is psychoanalytic and, as such, is usually discussed in comparison with earlier forms of psychoanalytic relational practice which have been developed since the inception of the profession including such notions as the so-called 'blank screen': see Hoffman (1983) for a comprehensive picture of this. Yet, in fact, the basic relational principles as practised today are fundamentally humanistic. The true beginnings of the movement can be found in Martin Buber's concept of I-Thou (1923) or Rudolf Steiner's view about relationship (1916) which are both inspired by spiritual world views but which go beyond the specifics of their own spiritual world view and become truly universal in a way which can go beyond any race, religion or belief. In spite of being a Rabbi in Hasidic Judaism Buber's ideas about dialogue are truly universal and in spite of being Christian in orientation Steiner's Anthroposophy is now seamlessly fitting well with Islam, Hinduism, Buddhism, Shinto and of course Judaism. They also share another important characteristic; namely that, in order to develop healthy relationships in the current age, we need to make great inner efforts. Buber speaks about making an effort in the I-Thou dialogue in order to develop awareness and respect for the other: 'each of the participants really has in mind the other or others in their present and particular being' (cited in Cissna & Anderson, 1998, p. 64). Steiner speaks about how we need to overcome our tendency today to meet other people in a 'far more impersonal manner' than we did in the past (Steiner, 1916, p. 119) in view of the fact that we are 'shut up in ourselves' (p. 120). We do this by 'paring down' our individuality when engaging with other people, reaching down into the depths of 'our own inner being' and applying 'inner development, inner activity' in our relationships (Steiner, 1916, p. 121).

In view of these factors it is not surprising that the relational turn now encompasses psychodynamic, humanistic and integrative approaches to healing (Loewenthal & Samuels, 2014). It has the potential, if fully recognized, to contribute to a balanced therapy profession in which the dominant IAPT intervention, cognitive behavioural therapy, is supplemented by these other therapies. They were, to some degree, in opposition to each other during the twentieth century (Lees, 2010). But the development of IAPT has already created a backlash which has prompted closer collaboration between these approaches to therapy, all of which are excluded from the IAPT evidence-based practice system. As illustrated in Loewenthal and Samuels' book they are now beginning to collaborate in regard to theory development, clinical technique and common social and political concerns.

There are several aspects to the relational turn which are relevant to this discussion. First, it adopts an approach to therapy based on mutuality in relationships rather than centralized managed care. Second, it sees the human being as a whole and does not just concentrate on parts of the human being; namely, symptoms. Third, it adopts a transformational approach to therapy rather than a resilience based approach. I will now look at these features.

Relationality rather than centralized management

Relational approaches to therapy see the field of interaction between the therapist and the client as a co-creation which is shaped by the inner worlds of both. Ideally, the relationship involves an intersubjective dyad of exploration and imagination (BCPSG, 2010) as opposed to the more traditional healing binary of healthy expert and ill patient which underpins IAPT and managed care. This produces a different sort of therapeutic relationship from the traditional doctor–patient or even psychotherapist–client dyad. Orbach (2014) uses the term 'democratic' to describe relational psychotherapy. It is a dynamic interaction between two subjectivities, both of whom have strengths and weaknesses, problems, pathologies, healthy aspects and who can 'diagnose' each other: 'Clinically, the most interesting aspect of the intersubjective environment between patient and analyst is the mutual knowing of what is on the other's mind, as it concerns the current nature and state of that relationship' (BCPSG, 2010, p. 7). The relationship is viewed as a matrix of interacting subjectivities which may 'include states of activation, affect, feeling, arousal, desire, belief, motive, or content of thought, in any combination' (ibid., p. 7) co-created by the therapist and the client.

Therapists participate in the work of co-creation and, in so doing, strive to establish a safe and trusting interpersonal field in which the potential of the relationship depends on the quality of the relationship itself rather than external protocols. Both participants can interact, be playful and creative in order to bring about a transformational healing process in ways that could not be anticipated at the outset in a predictive therapeutic protocol. The therapeutic relationship becomes a 'potential space' for change and transformation as originally described by Winnicott (Casement, 1985, p. 162). The intrapsychic state of mind of both the therapist and the client is affected, and developed, by the interactions between the two. These interactions can be broken down into a series of dialectical relationships which move between fantasy and reality (e.g. me and not-me, symbol and symbolized) in the minds of both of the participants in a way which informs and negates the views of each other (Ogden, 1985). This leads to a dynamic situation in which the therapist is constantly making new clinical judgements in response to the rapidly changing situation.

Relationality contrasts to the IAPT approach to care. Instead of emphasizing publicly accountable protocols and standardized evidence-based techniques, it emphasizes the private, intimate, complex and often intense and unpredictable ever-changing world of the therapist–client encounter and creative techniques. Instead of being backed up by large scale research studies, such as RCTs and meta analyses, it is based on research into the microphonema of the interaction (Seligman, 2012), which enables the interaction to be investigated in its holistic psychological, social and spiritual complexity and not just from the one-dimensional point of view of alleviating symptoms.

Holism rather than fragmentation

Managed care emphasizes 'recovery from' particular symptoms. In contrast relational approaches to therapy are based on the principle of 'recovery in' (Fisher & Lees, 2015). In the words of the epigraph to this chapter therapy 'starts from the position that there is no cure, but that we need different ways of living with ourselves and different descriptions of these so-called selves' as a result of the interaction. It is an approach to therapy based on holism rather than fragmentation. The limited focus on symptoms is progressively extended to include other phenomena.

The client's life story has been conceptualized in therapeutic research for many years in psychoanalysis, as Loewenthal reminds us (2014, p. 5), using such notions as the triangle of person (Malan, 1999). This provides a template for therapeutic work which goes far beyond the symptom. It links the relationship patterns displayed by the client in the presence of the therapist with relationships with other people and with people from the client's past. The therapeutic relationship is seen as a reflection of relationships from the client's life, past and present. In psychodynamic theory, as practised by intersubjective therapists, the immediate therapist–client relationship is linked with infant relationships. For instance, Stern's view about the transformational moments of meeting, a concept which I will return to later, is a timeless 'moment of meeting' which mirrors special moments in their infant relationships with a maternal figure as a result of verbal and non-verbal communication:

> the social smile emerges along with sustained mutual gaze and vocalization, the parent and baby amuse one another with facial and vocal exchanges. They are moving along. Then, something unpredictable happens (e.g., A funny facial expression or the unexpected vocal and facial synchronization, and all of a sudden they are laughing together). The interaction has been kicked up to a new and higher level of activation and joy that the baby may never before have achieved and which has never before been shared between them as an intersubjective context.
>
> *(Stern* et al.*, 1998, p. 305)*

Loewenthal (2014, p. 5) and many others, such as the contributors to this book, extend the holistic scope of the relationship further by looking at the relationship between the therapist and the client in a broader social and political context. Psychological problems are seen as meaningful responses to environmental and cultural stresses including the dominant ideas and the material conditions of the client's life and not just problems which are located in the individual in the form of a symptom (Fisher & Lees, 2015).

The holistic aspect of therapeutic work can be extended yet further in a way which integrates psychodynamic, humanistic, and even spiritual, principles. My preferred approach to clinical practice, anthroposophic psychotherapy, integrates all of these things. It brings together the psychological and the social with the somatic and the spiritual (Dekkers, 2015, Lees, 2011, 2015; Ritchie *et al.*, 2001). This includes, as in psychodynamic therapy, and attachment theory, the importance of early childhood. But it also looks at the whole life story or biography of the client. So healing involves understanding both the root of the problem in childhood, the issue of 'why now?' in terms of the current age of the client and the entirety of the client's unique life story (Burkhard, 1997; Lievegoed, 1979). It also encompasses both body and spirit: 'no so-called mental illness exists which is not accompanied by physical changes' and, on the other hand, 'psychological symptoms can help us to understand better what is taking place in the organism'

(Bott, 1978, p. 44). Finally, it incorporates health as well as illness; namely the principle of salutogenesis (Antonovsky, 1979) which supports health and well-being – 'salus' or health and 'genesis' or origin. It involves locating the client as located on a 'continuum on an axis between total ill health (dis-ease) and total health (ease)' (European Committee for Homeopathy *et al.*, 2008, p. 7). In humanistic terms it involves working with our healthy side and how we could be (our ego strength) as well as how we are. In view of these characteristics I call it a bio-psycho-social-spiritual approach to healing (Lees, 2013).

Transformation rather than resilience

In contrast to the managed care principle of building up resilience, the primary aim of relational holistic therapy is transformation of both symptoms and the whole human being. It is concerned with enabling the client to transform their lives in such a way that they can unfold their potential as opposed to just helping them to become resilient workers and consumers. We create a unique space between the therapist and client which aims to bring about mutual transformation as a result of 'exploring the gaps, or spaces between the therapist and client in the interaction and creating a space 'for the play of speculation' (Phillips, 1988). An important aspect of this space is the phenomenon of moments of meeting, or what Daniel Stern (2004) has also referred to as an experience of *kairos*:

> *Kairos* is the passing moment in which something happens as the time unfolds. It is the coming into being of a new state of things, and it happens in a moment of awareness. It has its own boundaries and escapes or transcends the passage of linear time. Yet it also contains a past. It is a subjective parenthesis set off from chronos. *Kairos* is a moment of opportunity, when events demand action or are propitious for action.
>
> *(Stern, 2004, p. 7)*

Such experiences open up the future as well as link our experience with the past as previously discussed. They bring about new possibilities (including new personal, social and political possibilities) as a result of the power of the meeting. Yet they go even further. They also take us into the eternal. Such an event 'has its own boundaries and escapes or transcends the passage of linear time' and yet is 'in some kind of dialogic equilibrium with the past and future' (Stern, 2004, p. 28). As a result of this they connect with the creative possibilities of the moment and the future.

Such moments are not confined to therapeutic work. They are also to be found in literature, biography and our everyday experience. As regards literature and biography several memorable meetings come to mind – the meeting between the Englishman, Fielding, and the Indian, Aziz, at the end of E. M. Forster's *Passage to India*, the meeting between Bertrand Russell and Joseph Conrad as described in Russell's autobiography (Symington, 1986) or the intense love between Virginia

Woolf and her sister, Vanessa Bell (Dunn, 2000). Whenever or wherever they occur they have the quality of both linear time and the eternal, can be meetings between people of the same, or different, genders, are passionate and express agape, rather than erotic, love. Moreover, they bring about new creative possibilities in the future. I would argue that they form an essential part of the creativity of all of the people involved: E. M. Forster, Bertrand Russell, Joseph Conrad, Virginia Woolf and Vanessa Bell.

Transformational moments enable us to affirm our existence in the physical world (body or soma), to connect with social life and our own life story (social and psychological). From the point of view of our individual experience they thus confirm our existence in spatial linear time. But they also unite us with our spiritual eternal existence. From the point of view of social life they provide the basis for overcoming the dominance of the neo-liberal market agenda in social life. We change ourselves in order to change the world. They free our spiritual eternal potential (Liberté) from the dominance of business thinking, help us to fully connect with social and political life (Égalité) as well as economic life and enable us to work harmoniously and cooperatively with each other as opposed to against each other in our economic relations (Fraternité). They help us to overcome the pervasive influence of the market.

The development of creative research methods

From the 1980s onwards, as managed care and evidence-based practice have developed, many new qualitative research methodologies have also developed in many of the human, social and clinical sciences – for instance, education, anthropology, sociology and nursing. They include such methodologies as autoethnography (Muncey, 2010), heuristic research (Moustakas, 1990), action research (McNiff & Whitehead, 1989) and narrative research (Richardson, 1994; Frank, 1995). They offer a naturalistic qualitative approach to research based on lived experience. In the field of counselling and psychotherapy they have been variously described as practitioner research (McLeod, 1999), learning by inquiry (Clarkson, 1998), reflexive action research (Lees, 2001), a non-procedural approach to research (Rennie, 2004) and practice-based research (Lees & Freshwater, 2008). The term that I am now using is transformational research.

The reason for using the term transformational research is threefold. First, it points to a close relationship between the transformational work undertaken by practitioners, especially counselling, psychotherapy and 'psychological therapy' practitioners, as opposed to the research undertaken by purely academic researchers or practitioners who are no longer engaged in practice. Second, as a result of this, it draws on the transferable skills which have been developed by practitioners and therapists in particular. Third, inasmuch as it is akin to therapeutic practice, and therapy practitioners are experts at doing it, it can reverse the direction of the usual trajectory of research. What I mean by this is that, whereas therapy practitioners have had to deal with research methods which have been imposed on them from the outside (that is to say they have been imported into the therapy profession from other disciplines), it opens up the possibility of research going in the opposite direction. In other words it is a research method which can be developed further by therapy practitioners and which they can then export to other professions.

It is beyond the scope of this chapter to discuss the method in detail. So, towards the end of this chapter, I will undertake a mini action research project to demonstrate how, utilizing these methods, it is possible to initiate a more constructive dialogue with advocates of managed care as opposed to the present stand-off. But, first, I will look at some of its major features. Its basic principles resemble relational therapy and thus, like relational therapy, counterbalance the principles of managed care which I have already discussed: centralized management control, a fragmentary approach to the human being based on symptoms and the emphasis on resilience.

Relationality rather than centralized management

One principle of good research is a standpoint of healthy scepticism with regard to one's own point of view (Robson, 2002). This provides a basis for enhancing our capacity to relate using the principle of reflexivity. Reflexivity can be defined in a number of ways. The definition I will adopt here is based on the notion of 'turning' or 'bending' something back on itself. Steier (1991, p. 2) refers to turning back 'one's experience upon oneself' while Freshwater and Rolfe (2001) discuss 'turning *thought* or *reflection* back on itself' and 'turning *action* or *practice* back on itself'. Therapists are familiar with these principles as a result of clinical supervision and their own personal therapy. It is similar to the notion of the internal supervisor (Casement, 1985) which we use in clinical supervision and our own reflections on practice.

Such research activity extends the relational views of Buber and Steiner; namely, that we need to make efforts to develop ourselves in order to truly engage in dialogue with others. In order to do this we reflexively examine our experience (and point of view) and turn it back on itself in a way which shows its limitations and flaws: we see the plank in our own eye rather than the mote in the eye of the other. Such an exercise then opens us up the possibility, in Buber's terms, of having 'in mind the other or others' or, in Steiner's terms, addressing the fact that we are 'shut up in ourselves' in the present age and find it difficult to go beyond our own views. So it emphasizes the importance of self-transformation in relationship.

Holism rather than fragmentation

The reflexive analytical process of transformational research, and its precursors, is cyclical and boundaryless (Lees, 2001, 2003) and thus, truly holistic. There are many aspects to this. It involves an ongoing process of cyclically and endlessly reflecting on experience in order to create new data. We thereby progressively expand the scope of the project to include all of the factors I mentioned in the previous section and develop a truly holistic perspective on the work including social and political life, our whole life story, the eternal, our body and our spirit. Put differently, 'the conventional boundaries between research, practical application and personal growth and transformation melt away' (Braud & Anderson, 1998, p. 43). Furthermore the boundary between researcher–respondent and therapist–client is also obscured (Lees, 2001, p. 135). Put differently, reflexivity destabilizes 'boundaries between me, my research and those with whom I engage in my research' (Maxey, 1999, p. 203). This resembles clinical work and in fact a piece of clinical work is also a research project. In clinical work, as in transformational research, we progressively expand our perspective on the work as we collect new data. We then analyse it, modify our perspective and start the cycle again. So transformational research resembles the transformational aspects of clinical practice. In clinical work the therapist and client are both affected by the process, usually in equal measure. In transformative research the researcher and the participants are both affected in exactly the same way. I will continue this theme in the next section.

Transformation rather than resilience

The main purpose of transformational research, and its antecedents, is, needless to say, to bring about transformation rather than to create resilient citizens to serve the needs of the State. Maxey (1999, p. 199) sees such research as having 'enormous liberatory potential' and says that 'by actively and critically reflecting on the world and our place within it, we are more able to act in creative, constructive ways that challenge oppressive power relations rather than reinforce them' (ibid., p. 201). It is about raising consciousness about the conditions of our lives: what Freire refers to as a process of 'conscientisation' (Freshwater, 2000, p. 26) and Mezirow refers to as 'perspective transformation' (Mezirow, 1981). As we engage in the cyclical iterative reflexive process, we are freed from the constraints of the resilience orientated market-driven anxieties and can see ever more clearly the conditions in which we are living and the way in which they affect our consciousness and state of mind. We are able to find ourselves and act freely (Liberté), recover our rights and human dignity (Egalité) and cooperate with other people in economic life (Fraternité).

The future of the profession

I will now, as discussed, engage in a mini research project to examine how the principles of relationality and transformational research can be applied in practice by using them to investigate the current state of affairs in the profession. I will begin with the hypothesis that, although managed care and evidence-based practice may at first seem to be incompatible with relational therapy and transformational research, it does not follow that they are unconnected or that a dialectical process of development between them is impossible. Perhaps, as Heraclitus says: 'there is an opposing coherence, as in the tensions of the bow and the lyre' (Geldard, 2000, p. 39).

In order to undertake this investigation I will use myself as a case study and examine my experience of IAPT and the development of the profession in the early years of the twenty-first century using the techniques of relational therapy and transformational research. In doing this I am using myself as a representative of the socialization and education we are all subject to in contemporary Western society and the effect that this has on us. There is of course a long tradition of therapists using themselves as case studies in our profession. In the 1890s, after the death of his father, Freud famously remarked that the case that most interested him was himself and, in the 1910s, after his break with Freud, Jung embarked on his inner journey of discovery as documented in *Memories, Dreams and Reflections*: a heuristic research project in which Jung examined his own inner life in depth and used it as a basis for developing the theories of analytical psychology.

My case study begins with the experience of teaching counselling and psychotherapy students. In so doing I do not hide my views and beliefs. I often set up a polarity between managed care and 'hard science' research methods, on the one hand, and relational practice and creative methodologies on the other. I have even written an article which highlights this polarity (Lees, 2005) and have done the same thing in this book. So here, too, I have set up a polarity. I have set the two points of view in binary opposition to each other. I have positioned each point of view in such a way as to be 'dependent on and contained within the other, so that neither is possible without the opposite' and have also ensured that 'one of them is seen as superior to the other' (Freshwater & Rolfe, 2004, p. 11); namely, my preference for relational psychotherapy and transformational research – for relational, holistic and transformational approaches to research and practice.

I will now examine my actions from the point of view of relational therapy and transformational research.

Relational therapy and my actions

As regards relationships it is helpful, once again, to remember the views of Buber and Steiner, namely, to make an effort in relationships today if they are to be healthy. I will do this by using the notion of the third. This is central to classical Freudian theory and builds on the theory of the Oedipus complex. To put it briefly the person who is able to tolerate rivalry in relationships, along with the possibility of being excluded from a union between the other two protagonists (i.e. tolerating a third), is more mature than the person who is in constant need of undivided and individual attention from another person and cannot tolerate such exclusion. This principle has been further developed in contemporary intersubjective relational theory and practice. Aron, basing his work on Benjamin, applies this principle to his clinical work in the notion of the 'third-in-the-one' whereby thirdness 'emerges within the dyad without needing a literal third object' (Aron, 2006, p. 358). He speaks about how, in situations of therapeutic impasse in the dyadic relationship, the therapist may create a third by disclosing 'their own inner conflict and self-disagreement' (ibid., p. 359) with comments such as 'I'm in two minds about this' or 'part of me thinks this and part of me thinks that' or 'I have this sense that you are saying that but maybe I'm wrong'.

My undeveloped perspective on the profession is essentially dyadic and, holding this position, I am creating an impasse as a result of my tendency to polarize the dyad and set up binaries in which I place relational practice and transformative research in a superior position to managed care and evidence-based practice. Again this is a characteristic which I find difficult to avoid as a result of my socialization and education in contemporary Western society. In order to move on from this I need to bring in a third without, as Aron says, 'a literal third object'. To some degree I have already begun to do this by questioning the dyad itself and bringing to my consciousness my 'own inner conflict and self-disagreement' with my tendency to polarize and set up binaries. I am thereby adopting a relational and dialogical position which involves deconstructing my own point of view.

Transformational research and my perspective

I will now subject my standpoint to transformational research analysis; that is to say, I will reflexively turn my thoughts and reflections back on themselves. This enables me to raise my level of consciousness and develop a fuller, more holistic view of my actions. First, I become aware that, in putting together this book, I contradict myself. On the one hand, I am espousing a balanced profession in which the two positions are in dialogue with each other and, on the other, I am setting the different positions in opposition with each other. Second, I have logically analysed the written material to bring order into the book and in what I write to make sure that the thoughts systematically flow from one another. (Whether I achieve this or not is another matter.) This action utilizes systematization and logic. I want to impose something on the situation because, if I did not do this, I would drown in a stream of consciousness. Third, I extend this principle to my therapy work. There, too, I can sometimes be systematic, logical and driven by theoretical 'protocols' rather than seeing the reality in front of my eyes. So when I am critiquing the clinical principles underpinning IAPT, I am actually critiquing part of myself (there's a bit of IAPT manager or practitioner in me). Fourth, I accept that we are living and working at a time when everything is quantified and measured, where 'counting and formulaic approaches to research have been and continue to some extent to hold the position of a dominant discourse' (Freshwater, 2014) and it is inevitable that I am affected by this. Part of me wants to be 'formulaic, robotic, disembodied' and wants to adopt 'objective modes of defining, categorizing, predicting, and boxing certain types of research questions everything to be the same and repeatable' (ibid.) even in my practice. At some level I want everything to be the same. It is so much easier.

The profession today and in the future

In this mini research project I have clarified how I am influenced by internalized discourses, including the discourses which I find unpalatable simply by virtue of the fact that a way of thinking has been inculcated into me by my socialization and education. As a result of examining this from the point of view of relational practice and transformational research principles I can see how this can create problems and contradictions. In so doing I am able to expand my perspective on my actions – and we all have the possibility of doing this. Such an inner effort then enhances our capacity to constructively engage with different points of view even if they are different from our own. As regards the topic of this discussion such engagement can contribute to taking the profession forward in spite of the challenges it is facing. It enables us to become more conscious of the social conditions which have shaped us. We are then in a stronger position to strip away the dross created by internalized discourses in the sense of Foucauldian discourse analysis (Willig, 2001) and take actions in the world based on our 'own value system' (Dekkers, 2015). It is concerned with making both our limitations (what is holding us back) and our true values transparent. In my case I am then able to act out of my desire to be as inclusive as possible. In Jungian terms it is an essential part of individuation which includes confronting our shadow – or what, in anthroposophic psychotherapy is referred to as the double (Lievegoed, 1985).

Becoming conscious of our values is important and significant. According to Nuttall (2015), citing the work of Gordon Allport, there are six categories of values – economic, aesthetic, social, political, spiritual and scientific. Applying these principles to this discussion is illuminating. Managed care is based on economic, conventional scientific and centralized political values while I, as a practitioner, base my work on aesthetic, social and spiritual values. I am sure that the proponents of IAPT think that, in the light of their values, their cause is right just as those of us who have 'practitioner' values think that our cause is right. Moreover I imagine that we hold on to these different positions with equal passion and conviction. I take the view that the mind set of IAPT poses many problems for the future of our profession – and society at large – and those who hold 'IAPT' values no doubt think that my position is equally questionable.

The main problem is how these different values can meet. Merely becoming conscious of the differences in values does not in itself take the profession forward. A key value in my work is my spiritual values (and here I am thinking about spirituality in the broadest sense of the term which can be held by anyone whether we hold to an overtly spiritual or religious world view or not). For me this relates to the inner developmental process which requires effort and which I have already described. In order to reach my core values I need to engage in a rigorous process of self-development aided by relational therapy and creative research methods in order to see the limits of my own point of view. Indeed Nuttall (2015) says the same thing in a different way. He refers to the fact of developing the four qualities of individuation, including knowing our own shadow, aspiration, solicitude and congruence. Such a developmental process reflects the quintessence of therapeutic activity. It involves, quoting Ogden again, engaging in a 'series of dialectical relationships which move between fantasy and reality' – in this case with myself.

Whichever way we look at the situation facing us in the therapy profession today I believe we possess the tools to respond to the problems and challenges facing us based on its transformative principles. We can, for instance, adopt an overriding integrative and inclusive approach to them, at least within ourselves. This is similar to Gandhi's notion of Satyagraha. It gives us the basis for meaningful dialogue and effective action.

Note

1   I want to acknowledge the contribution of my colleague, Dr Pamela Fisher, to this article. Her ideas about the social and political context of managed care and the principle of resilience started the process. We then co-authored an article on this theme. Finally, I used it as the starting point for this chapter.

References

Antonovsky, A. (1979). *Health, stress and coping*. San Francisco, CA: Jossey-Bass.

Aron, L. (2014). Relational psychotherapy in Europe: A view from across the Atlantic. In D. Loewenthal & A. Samuels (eds), *Relational Psychotherapy, Psychoanalysis and Counselling* (pp. 93–106). London: Routledge.

BCPSG. (2010). *Change in psychotherapy: A unifying paradigm*. London: W. W. Norton.

Bott, V. (1978). *Anthroposophical medicine*. London: Rudolf Steiner Press.

Braud, W. & Anderson, R. (1998). Conventional and expanded views of research. In W. Braud & R. Anderson (eds), *Transpersonal research methods for the social sciences* (pp. 3–26). Thousand Oaks, CA: Sage.

Buber, M. (1923). I and Thou. In W. Herberg (ed.), *The writings of Martin Buber*. Cleveland, OH: Meridian Books.

Burkhard, G. (1997). *Taking charge*. Edinburgh, UK: Floris Books.

Casement, P. (1985). *On learning from the patient*. London: Tavistock.

Cissna, K. N. & Anderson, R. (1998). Theorizing dialogic moments: The Buber-Rogers position and postmodern times. *Communicative Theory*, 8(1), 63–104.

Clarkson, P. (1998). Learning through Inquiry (the Dierotao programme at PHYSIS). In P. Clarkson (ed.), *Counselling psychology: Integrating theory, research and supervised practice*. London: Routledge.

Dekkers, A. (2015). *The psychotherapy of human dignity*. Soon to be published in English.

Dunn, J. (2000). *Virginia Woolf and Vanessa Bell*. London: Virago.

European Committee for Homeopathy, European Council of Doctors for Plurality in Medicine, International Council of Medical Acupuncturists and Related Techniques, International Federation of Anthroposophical Medical Associations. (2008). *Complementary Medicine (CAM): Its current position and its potential for European healthcare*. Brussels and Strasburg: Joint Report.

Fisher, P. & Lees, J. (2015). Narrative and mental health: Preserving the emancipatory tradition. *Under peer review*.

Frank, A. W. (1995). *The wounded storyteller*. Chicago, IL: The University of Chicago Press.

Freshwater, D. (2000). *Transformatory learning in nurse education*. Southsea, UK: Nursing Praxis International.

Freshwater, D. (2014). What counts in mixed methods research: Algorithmic thinking or inclusive leadership? *Journal of Mixed Methods Research*, 8, 327.

Freshwater, D. & Rolfe, G. (2001). Critical reflexivity: A politically and ethically engage research method for nursing. *NT Research*, 6(1), 526–37.

Freshwater, D. & Rolfe, G. (2004). *Deconstructing evidence-based practice.* London: Routledge.

Geldard, R. G. (2000). *Remembering Heraclitus.* Edinburgh, UK: Floris Books.

Herman, J. (1992). *Trauma and recovery.* New York: Basic Books.

Hoffmann, I. Z. (1983). The patient's experience of the analyst's experience. *Contemporary Psychoanalysis, 19,* 389–422.

Humphries, J. (2015). Interview. A history of Britain in numbers. *BBC Radio,* 4, 23 February 2015. Retrieved on 25 February 2015 from: www.bbc.co.uk/programmes/b053721c.

Layard, R. (2006). *The depression report: A new deal for depression and anxiety disorders.* London: London School of Economics.

Lees, J. (2001). Reflexive action research: Developing knowledge through practice. *Counselling and Psychotherapy Research, 1*(2), 132–8.

Lees, J. (2003). Developing therapist self-understanding through research. *Counselling and Psychotherapy Research, 3*(2), 147–53.

Lees, J. (2005). Two research discourses. *Therapy Today, 16*(8), 29–31.

Lees, J. (2010). Identity wars, the counselling and psychotherapy profession and practitioner-based research. *Psychotherapy and Politics International, 8*(1), 3–12.

Lees, J. (2011). Counselling and psychotherapy in dialogue with complementary and alternative medicine. *British Journal of Guidance and Counselling, 39*(2), 117–30.

Lees, J. (2013). Psychotherapy, complementary and alternative medicine and social dysfunction. *European Journal of Psychotherapy and Counselling, 15*(3), 201–3.

Lees, J. (2015). Psychosomatics and physical and psychological trauma. *Under peer review.*

Lees, J. & Freshwater, D. (eds) (2008). *Practitioner-based research: Power, discourse and transformation.* London: Karnac Books.

Lievegoed, B. (1979). *Phases.* London: Rudolf Steiner Press.

Lievegoed, B. (1985). *Man on the threshold.* Stroud, UK: Hawthorn Press.

Loewenthal, D. (2014). The magic of the relational? An introduction to appraising and reappraising relational psychotherapy, psychoanalysis and counselling. In D. Loewenthal & A. Samuels (eds), *Relational psychotherapy, psychoanalysis and counselling* (pp. 184–92). London: Routledge.

Loewenthal, D. & Samuels, A. (eds) (2014). *Relational psychotherapy, psychoanalysis and counselling.* London: Routledge.

Malan, D. (1999). *Individual psychotherapy and the science of psychodynamics.* Oxford: Butterworth-Heimann.

McLeod, J. (1999). *Practitioner research in counselling.* London: Sage.

McNiff, J., Lomax, P. & Whitehead, J. (1989). *You and your action research project.* London: Routledge.

Maxey, I. (1999). Beyond boundaries? Activism, academia, reflexivity and research. *Area, 31*(3), 199–208.

Mezirow, J. (1981). A critical theory of adult learning and education. *Adult Education, 32,* 3–24.

Moustakas, C. (1990). *Heuristic research: Methodology and application.* London: Sage.

Muncey, T. (2010). *Creating autoethnographies.* London: Sage.

NHS. (2015). Guidance on new mental health standards published. Downloaded on 20 March from: www.england.nhs.uk/2015/02/13/mh-standards/.

Nuttall, J. (2015). Getting values across – Leadership in a multi-cultural world. Chancellor's Invitation Lecture, 6 May 2014. London: Regent's University London.

O'Brien, N. (2013). The remarkable rise of mental illness in Britain. Dowloaded on 26 September 2013 from: http://blogs.telegraph.co.uk/news/neilobrien1/100186974/the-remarkable-rise-of-mental-illness-in-britain/.

Ogden, T. H. (1985). On potential space. *The International Journal of Psychoanalysis, 66*(2), 129–41.

Orbach, S. (2014). Democratizing psychoanalysis. In D. Loewenthal & A. Samuels (eds), *Relational psychotherapy, psychoanalysis and counselling* (pp. 12–26). London: Routledge.

Phillips, A. (1988). *Winnicott*. London: Fontana Paperbacks.

Rennie, D. L. (2004). Anglo-North American qualititative counselling and psychotherapy research. *Psychotherapy Research, 14*(1), 37–55.

Richardson, L. (1994). Writing as a method of inquiry. In N. K. Denzin & Y. S. Lincoln (eds), *Handbook of Qualitative research*. London: Sage.

Ritchie, J., Wilkinson, J., Gantley, M., Feder, G., Carter, Y. & Formby, J. (2001). *A model of integrated primary care: Anthroposophic medicine*. London: University of London.

Roberts, J. M. (2004). John Stuart Mill, free speech and the public sphere: A Bakhtinian critique. *The Sociological Review, 52*(s1), 67–87.

Robson, C. (2002). *Real world research*. Oxford: Blackwell.

Seligman, S. (2012). The baby out of the bathwater: Microseconds, psychic structure and psychotherapy. *Psychoanalytic Dialogues, 22*, 499–509.

Sennett, R. (1998). *The corrosion of character*. London: W. W. Norton.

Steier, F. (1991). Introduction: research as self-reflexivity, self-reflexivity as process. In F. Steier (ed.), *Research and reflexivity*. London: Sage.

Steiner, R. (1916/1999). *The meaning of life*. London: Rudolf Steiner Press.

Steiner, R. (1923/1977). *Towards social renewal*. London: Rudolf Steiner Press.

Stern, D. N., Bruschweiler-Stern, N., Harrison, A. M., Lyons-Ruth, K., Morgan, A. C., Nahum, J. P., Sander, L. W. & Tronick, E. Z. (1998). The process of therapeutic change involving implicit knowledge: Some implications of developmental observations for adult psychotherapy. *Infant Mental Health Journal, 19*(3), 300–8. doi: 10.1002/(sici)1097-0355(199823)19:3<300::aid-imhj5>3.0.co;2-p.

Stern, D. N. (2004). *The present moment in psychotherapy and everyday life*. New York: W. W. Norton.

Symington, N. (1986). *The analytic experience*. London: Free Association Books.

Willig, C. (2001). *Qualitative research in psychology*. Maidenhead, UK: Open University Press.

10

THE RISK-TAKING PResENTITIONER

THE RISK-TAKING PRACTITIONER

Implementing freedom in clinical practice

Nick Totton

> He [sic] who is subject to a field of visibility, and knows it, assumes responsibility
> for the constraints of power, he makes them play spontaneously upon himself; he
> inscribes in himself the power relations in which he simultaneously plays both
> roles, he becomes the principle of his own subjection.
>
> *(Foucault, 1977, pp. 202–3)*

Introduction

Over recent years there has been an enormously powerful trend towards making
the practice of psychotherapy and counselling (hereinafter usually 'therapy') safe.
This has included lengthening trainings; making assessment and accreditation
more rigorous; developing evidence-based practice; collecting client assessment;
elaborating complaint procedures and much more. This has amounted to the
installation, on the practice of therapy, of a surveillance culture, partly external
and partly – as Foucault indicates in the epigraph to this chapter – internal.

Much of this worthy endeavour, however, has been more or less a waste
of time, because it is based on a complete misunderstanding of what sort of
activity therapy is. Like life, therapy is inherently risky. Like people's lives, no two
therapies – let alone two therapists – are the same; and as with life, although many
interesting views can be expressed about the best way to do therapy, none of them
can be rigorously demonstrated to be true. Therapy is not a medical practice, but
a practice of truth; hence measures of efficacy and effectiveness are at cross purposes
to its project. Furthermore, internal and external surveillance is precisely what most
clients are in one way or another suffering from when they arrive; to install the
process within the therapy room, therefore, virtually guarantees the failure of therapy.

The statements made in the previous paragraph are interconnected and inter-
dependent; I am now going to develop each of them separately, while trying to

show the links between them. I will look at therapy as risk, the fact that no two therapies are the same, the difficulty in demonstrating that one is truer than another and thus the best therapeutic practice, therapy as the practice of truth, and the problems of surveillance. I will then conclude the chapter by looking at a way forward for the profession.

Therapy is inherently risky

> Risk taking is as unavoidable in therapy as it is in life.
>
> *(Bond, 2006, p. 84)*

It should be immediately clear that if the statement above is true, then all practitioners are risk-takers; it's just a matter of whether we know it or not. I shall be arguing that conscious and deliberate risk taking is in fact an ethical requirement, and the only way to mitigate the dangers of unconscious risk taking.

I'm pleased to be able to lead off this section with a quotation from Tim Bond, because he is largely responsible for giving credibility to current approaches to professional ethics, particularly within BACP. Yet somehow his many sophisticated and realistic theoretical contributions on these issues end up being operationalised as crass, simplistic and authoritarian codes of practice. I have no idea how this happens or how Bond feels about it, but if it were me, I would be very frustrated.

I suspect, however, that he is perhaps more responsible than he may realise for this degradation of his theories in practice. There are subtle flaws in Bond's work, neatly encapsulated in this passage:

> I think it is realistic to expect ethics that are primarily designed to inform and support practice to have the following characteristics: . . . Simple enough to be both readily recalled by busy practitioners during the course of their work and readily communicable to others, including clients.
>
> *(Bond, 2006, p. 78)*

Are ethics something to be 'readily recalled'? And – even worse in my view – are they something that we can afford to simplify *just in order* for them to be easy to remember? This surely implies that they are a set of instructions we have received passively from an external source. But this understanding of ethics turns them into *laws*, which I would argue represent a wholly different concept. We obey laws either to avoid punishment, or because we have a prior – ethical – principle that we *should* obey laws. But we follow ethical principles because we believe them to be right; and belief, in this context, is not something centred in our reason, and certainly not centred in *someone else's* reason, but something we experience as an embodied sense of 'rightness' about one course of action and 'wrongness' about another one.

Real ethics are in our bones – an implicit knowledge (Boston Change Process Study Group, 2008) which, on later examination, will turn out to have motivated our actions whether we were consciously thinking about it or not. In fact, sometimes it is through our instinctive actions that we discover an ethical position in ourselves of which we were previously unaware. I am thinking of the scene in *In Treatment: Series 1* (Garcia, 2008) where the Gabriel Byrne character goes to see a recent ex-client, fully intending to have sex with her: they get as far as the bedroom – then everything goes blank and he finds himself outside the building, dazed and shocked. His body has made an ethical decision, while his head was still busy trying to justify making a mistake.

Over the past decades, however, there has been an increasing tendency for discussions of so-called 'professional ethics' to actually be about rules, about laws; talking to trainees and recent graduates of trainings, most of them do this quite unselfconsciously, because they have been taught that this is what ethics *means* – essentially, avoiding getting into trouble: defensive practice. There are a number of reasons for this shift, including changes in the cultural context in which we operate, and I will return to some of these; but there are also brutally practical issues involved – trainees, who may not even be really suited for the work in terms of personal character and life experience, are being invited to take on difficult and demanding clients, without being paid, long before they have had the opportunity to discover a meaningful professional ethics.

In these circumstances, essentially financially driven, it is not surprising that trainers and supervisors resort to crude 'Thou shalt not' instructions – 'simple enough.' as Bond says 'to be readily recalled' – in an attempt to avoid the most egregious errors that inevitably arise from this situation: the equivalent of saying 'Don't point a loaded gun at anyone' and hoping for the best. The real ethical failure, it seems to me, is in the current mode of organisation of training and therapy provision which puts trainees and new graduates in this unfair situation.

However the 'Thou shalt not' approach is not restricted to this sort of context – essentially, an emergency. In one of many examples in our profession of the tail wagging the dog, it is generalised to the practice even of the most experienced. One effect of this ethical failure is that it discourages practitioners from exploring the true therapeutic value of risk; the 'Therapy Police' (Totton, 2010) installed in their heads press the alarm button and the practitioner backs off, even when they know that boundary-crossing (as distinct from boundary-violation: Gutheil & Gabbard, 1993) would be best for the client. At the same time as this ethical dumbing down is happening, however, it has become widely acknowledged that a major driving force in therapeutic change is the development of an authentic relationship between client and therapist. But how is authentic relationship possible without risk – of misunderstanding, of breach of trust, of failure? The concept of *enactment* is becoming more and more widely recognised – that past trauma needs to reappear, take flesh and blood form, within the therapy room, in order to stand a chance of being resolved (Maroda, 2002). But how can there be enactment without risk? Enactment will happen whether we are conscious of it or not, but it is far less risky when we *are* conscious and accepting.

Tim Bond says it very clearly:

> To be totally risk avoidant is to be ineffective and to collude with existing patterns that have become problematic. . . . Risk and uncertainty are inescapable existential challenges that face all therapists and their clients, and . . . they are often only partially and inadequately addressed in existing approaches to ethics.
>
> *(Bond, 2006, p. 78)*

However, this partiality and inadequacy continues in the BACP Ethical Framework which Bond was deeply involved in creating (BACP, 2012, 2013); and it becomes much worse in the current BACP proposals for a new version of the framework (BACP, 2014).

The paper of Bond's (Bond, 2006) from which I have been quoting implicitly justifies this by distinguishing between new and inexperienced therapists who need a firm structure of rules, and experienced therapists who can manage appropriate risk taking (not a distinction which is really made in the BACP Ethical Framework). But there are problems with this. First, rather like a religious cult, it sets up an inner circle, a 'we' who share the true picture, as opposed to an outer circle, 'they' who are fed a falsely simplified picture. And second, as I have already suggested, it is not clear how someone can move from the outer to the inner circle without gaining experience in risk taking.

No two therapies or therapists are the same

The title of this section is not intended to refer to *therapeutic modalities* – though that is clearly true – but to individual courses of therapy between a particular client and therapist. Real life therapy 'in the wild', so to speak, is composed of one-time-only events. The practitioners may approach all their clients with the same therapeutic principles in mind; but how those principles unpack and express themselves in contact with each particular client is unique and distinctive. There is a real parallel with gene expression: the new science of epigenetics studies the ways in which different genes from the genome come to be utilised in response to environmental circumstances, so that the same basic toolkit can be embodied in a huge variety of ways.

At most, therefore, we could visualise a particular therapist equipped with an implicit and highly complex decision tree when meeting a new client: 'If a, then x, if b then y . . . ' carried to the ultimate degree of possible variation, so that by the time the interaction has moved through several stages there may be little apparent relationship between one branch of the tree and another one. But although the process could possibly in principle be modelled in this way, this is of course not what the practitioner is *experiencing* as she works. It is hard to observe the internal process as it is going on; but if I try to think about my own experience, it seems that when I am with a client I enter a state of relaxed spontaneity, where I am not attempting to follow any programme, but allowing responses to arise in me as freshly as possible: responses which I then turn this way and that in my hands, considering carefully before deciding whether to offer them to the client or whether to feed them back into the pool of information which is guiding my understanding.

But even this process of consideration is not, in the first instance at least, really theoretically based. It feels much more like testing a bell or a glass by tapping gently to see whether it gives back a clear tone. I am testing my response for resonance. Theory only consciously comes in as one possible sort of spontaneous response: in the presence of a client I often find myself thinking about some particular concept or model, and experience tells me that this will usually turn out, though perhaps not immediately, to offer helpful insight into the client's process. I read widely about therapy and counselling, and there are several theoretical structures which are familiar enough for me to make use of them in this way; I often recommend to trainees and supervisees that they get to know a minimum of two modalities in this way – and using more than one model of course guarantees a wide range of possible therapeutic processes. But I agree with Arnold Mindell (Mindell, 1985, pp. 8–9) that prior theory is not essential: through working accurately with a client's process and with our responses to it, we could spontaneously 'rediscover' any existing form of therapy. Of course, it might save time to read a few books!

My general point, though, is that every course of therapy is uniquely constructed from the encounter between a particular therapist, with all her personal history, therapeutic experience and theoretical knowledge, and a particular client, with all *her* personal history, life experience, and theories about how things work. As I have written elsewhere (Totton, 2011), the therapy room is in fact a place where not just individuals but whole *networks* encounter each other, represented by the therapist and the client – networks that extend through time and space via relationships of family, of work, of friendship and identification. The same thing is equally true when any two people meet – it's true of you and your dentist – and the manualised approach to therapy indeed seeks to make it as similar as possible to seeing the dentist. Ironically, however, not even seeing the dentist is a fully manualised experience – there is a great deal of room for variation, for individual choice; and therapy is an activity where the individual variation *is* the work, where what in dentistry might perhaps be seen as the bits around the edge of good professional practice actually hold centre stage.

It is not possible to identify a best therapeutic practice

This next point follows directly from the previous one: if each therapeutic encounter is, *and needs to be*, unique, then little can be established about what should happen – beyond saying that it should follow the unique needs of the situation and respect the client's human rights. I must emphasise that this does not mean there is no place for talking and writing about how to do therapy! I spend a good deal of my time engaged in these activities, and listening to or reading others who are doing the same. But these ideas are just that, ideas, not conclusions: interesting, sometimes illuminating and inspiring, but unprovable – there can be no experimental verification where each encounter is unique.

No two clients have identical issues, and no two courses of therapy, even with the same practitioner, go in identical directions; while the goal in relation to which the effectiveness of the therapy might be assessed is often defined very differently *after* the work than *before,* by both the client and the practitioner: sometimes part of the therapy is realising that one's initial goals were misconceived. Attempts to bypass these problems by manualising therapy are, not to put too fine a point on it, farcical. The whole quixotic effort to answer unanswerable questions about 'what works' is fuelled by accountancy, and can be rephrased as 'What is the smallest number of sessions with the cheapest practitioner that we can get away with?'

The answer to this unfortunate question depends entirely on what we think we are trying to do. Are we trying to offer someone the possibility of exploring their life choices up to now and into the future, and the thoughts and feelings that go with them, in the company of an experienced and interested partner? Or are we trying to suppress their unpleasant symptoms and get them back to work? Or – and personally I think this is probably the best choice – are we entering into relationship with them with an openness to *their* wants and needs, and a willingness to offer either our help in meeting them or a referral to someone better suited?

You may notice that I have moved from the accountancy question to a series of options addressed to the practitioner themselves. And this is very much to the point: it is becoming increasingly hard for anyone except the self-employed therapist to ask these questions and explore these options. What is noticeable is how ideology follows economics – the less money there is available for long term therapy which allows exploration in depth, the more theories pop up which justify short term work, justify manualisation, treat practitioners as interchangeable so that the client's lack of choice appears unimportant. And it is not only management and commissioning bodies who take on these convenient theories: the practitioners themselves are increasingly becoming hypnotised into believing them.

Therapy is not medicine, but a practice of truth

> Many critics have suggested that the rise of neurobiology is leading to a kind of reductionism in which mental states are reduced to brain states, human actions are generated by brains rather than conscious individuals, and the key dimensions of our humanness – language, culture, history, society – are ignored. . . . For some, this rests on a philosophical error: attributing to brains capacities that can only properly be attributed to people . . . For others, it is the apotheosis of contemporary individualism – a turn away from social context to a vision of society as an aggregate of isolated individuals.
>
> *(Rose & Abi-Rached, 2013, pp. 20–1)*

That therapy is not a medical practice seems to many people obvious beyond argument. After all, despite numerous attempts there is not one psychological state for which a physical etiology has been convincingly demonstrated (Bentall, 2010) – yes, correlations with brain activity can be seen, as with any emotional state, but correlation is not cause. Hence the term 'mental illness' is inappropriate, based on the combination of a crude materialism with an equally crude political correctness – to call someone 'ill' seems somehow more acceptable than to call them mad or unhappy or anxious or in emotional pain. We all 'know' that the appropriate treatment for an illness is symptomatic relief: we find a medicine or a physical procedure which removes the experience being complained of, and call it a job well done.

But what I think prevents therapy from throwing off this ill-fitting socio-philosophical clothing is – as so often – an economic factor. Therapy has thrown in its lot with the NHS, partly so that psychotherapists and counsellors can get jobs, and partly, more altruistically, so that clients can get therapy without having to pay for it at the point of delivery. (NHS treatment is not free, but paid for out of taxation and National Insurance.)

The price of this arrangement for therapy has turned out to be very high – and in hindsight, inevitable. If therapy is an NHS treatment, then it is by definition medical; and if it is medical, then it must be evidence-based – and what counts as evidence for our views about good and effective practice is not our experience of working with many clients over many years, but a quite different yardstick which is taken to be more 'objective'. This is generally either a statistical treatment of a large group of clients who can be regarded as all having the 'same' problem (because it is given the same name) and be treated in the 'same' way – ideally through randomised control trials; or else an application to the therapeutic context of some finding from 'hard' science, mainly neuroscience.

The quote marks in the previous paragraph represent a condensed critique of this theory of evidence, a critique which it would take up too much space to spell out in full. (I have written about these issues at more length in Totton, 2012; see also Postle, 2007; House & Totton, 2011.) The positivist notion of objectivity which informs the statistical approach is both questionable in itself and wholly inapplicable to psychotherapy, whereas we have already seen meaningful definitions of effectiveness are extremely hard to come by. Neuroscience, however, raises more complex issues altogether: ultimately, one of cultural hegemony. What I observe in current writing about both body psychotherapy and psychotherapy in general is an enormous overvaluation of the contribution that neuroscience can make to our work. This in turn stems, I think, from a massive misunderstanding of how neuroscience and psychotherapy relate to each other – which in turn rests on a misunderstanding about how brain, body, environment and mind relate to each other.

There are probably several causes for this state of affairs; for body psychotherapists, certainly, an important factor has been an enormous strengthening of our own status in the psychotherapy world through the almost dreamlike confirmation given by neuroscience to many of our most treasured insights, which I will discuss below. But the central and most obvious cause is clearly the unique status claimed by and assigned to science in our culture. Nikolas Rose and Joelle Abi-Rached are very clear about how this status affects our reception of neuroscience's findings:

> Despite the well-known technical problems, assumptions, and limitations of these technologies, and the fact that they do not speak for themselves and must be interpreted by experts, the images have undoubted powers of persuasion, and their apparent ability to track mental processes objectively, often processes outside the awareness of the individual themselves, have proved persuasive in areas from neuromarketing to policies on child development.
> *(Rose & Abi-Rached, 2013, p. 13)*

I would substitute for the medical model of psychotherapy and counselling a model of therapy as *the practice of truth* (Totton, 2004). We live in a culture where systematic lying, without either remorse or consequences, is more and more a normal part of public life. Therapy is intrinsically concerned with truth and untruth and their respective consequences. This could be said of several other practices; but unlike the science of philosophy, the truth it studies is not only, or even mainly, rational but also emotional; and unlike religion, it asserts, truthfully, that there is no absolute, singular truth, but only plural and contingent truths, subject to negotiation. The move away from absolute truth is the greatest achievement of modernity, and therapy is wholly identified with it – apart from the superficial accretions of positivism which I have been describing.

Surveillance is what clients already suffer from

The massive rise in surveillance and monitoring which therapists have experienced over recent years is in many ways only a minor by-blow of the way in which these factors have become central in our whole culture since – to pick a convenient but approximate landmark – the events of 9/11 (Lyon, 2003, 2004). In fact, anti-terrorist hypervigilance is only half the story here: it has dovetailed neatly with a more gradually intensifying emphasis on the themes of *safety* and *blame*. Everything that happens in our world must be safe; and if it turns out not to be, this must be someone's fault.

This fantasy is conveniently neat and satisfying when applied to some aspects of life; but it gets into great difficulties when applied either to aspects which are intrinsically unsafe, or to aspects where there is a concealed social requirement that they be unsafe. Therapy is inescapably bound up with both of these. Its focus on relationships and feelings opens up the inherent riskiness of life, which I have already referred to; and also the ways in which we are put at risk by the ways in which life in late capitalism is structured.

These aspects of therapy make it a social irritant, as is pretty clear from the difficulty that our culture has in 'placing' therapy and therapists (Totton, 2008): it tends to look to us to provide 'cures' for ills which it is unable or unwilling to resolve – child sexual abuse, say, or antisocial behaviour – in both cases one segment of society focuses on punishment, another on therapy or counselling, but neither is prepared to face the deep social, economic and political issues involved. Therapists are supposed to smooth away people's pain at being unemployed, being treated in racist or sexist ways, being old and ignored. No wonder it has been called – for completely different reasons – the impossible profession (Malcolm, 2011)!

The imaginary power to cure social ills which therapy is granted goes alongside an imaginary power to do harm. Because our power to 'see through' people is exaggerated (to the extent that people at parties run away from us, in case we expose their deepest frailties), we are regarded as capable of Svengali-like manipulation, seduction, destruction of clients' autonomy and will. Therefore we have to be *watched* – subjected to Jeremy Bentham's Panopticon (Foucault, 1977), a CCTV camera in the corner of the therapy room ceiling, ready to alert the Therapy Police to break down the door and drag us off to Azkaban.

But wait, there is no Panopticon! The Therapy Police are (mostly) in our own heads, it is internally that they do their most damaging work, nudging us into defensive practice – working in a particular way not because it feels to us best for the client, but because it feels best for *us* and is least likely to get us into trouble with our professional body. We are so busy watching our backs that it is hard to attend to the client in front of us, what they are saying or what they need from us.

And with tragic irony, what they so often need from us is a space free from their own Panopticon, their own internal surveillance, the inner critic installed in childhood. They come to therapy suffering from enormous perceived demands on them to *be good*, even perfect; to make no mistakes, commit no sins, have no inappropriate thoughts or desires. They have inside them the bigger cousin of the Therapy Police – Life Police. One aspect of what therapy is for, it seems to me, is to help clients realise that their internal surveillance system is actually imaginary: that Big Brother is not watching them from the inside, even if he is alive and well on the outside. This realisation allows a huge relaxation to take place, which makes a space in which many problems can be solved.

But how can we help clients dismantle their internal surveillance system when we are at the mercy of our own? How can we support them in being spontaneous when we are double-checking everything we do against a 'readily recalled' list of instructions? How can we create a space for taking life-enhancing risks when we are ourselves terrified of being caught out and punished?

Is there a way forward?

I have written elsewhere that the opposite pole to the one-sided concept of 'therapeutic boundaries' is, not *boundarilessness*, but *boundlessness* – thinking of the connotations of the term in Buddhist thinking.

Undefensive practice, I suggest, draws on a sense of boundlessness – abundance, space, attention, care. In contact with abundance, a therapist can afford to be generous on many levels.

(Totton, 2010, p. 70)

I have conducted workshops based on this paper a number of times around the country, to experienced therapists and to trainees. It is probably the most successful workshop I have done, and has always been received with great enthusiasm. Practitioners are hungry for a sense of generous abundance rather than the sort of meanness that stems from scarcity. We need it, and our clients need it even more; without it, effective therapy is more or less impossible. I ended that paper with two sentences I cannot improve on:

Yes, a therapist who cannot offer her clients boundaries is dangerous. But a therapist who cannot offer her clients boundlessness is useless.

(Totton, 2010, p. 70)

References

BACP (2012). *Statement of ethical practice.* Lutterworth, UK: BACP.

BACP (2013). *The ethical framework for good practice in counselling,* rev. edn. Lutterworth, UK: BACP.

BACP (2014). *Ethical framework for the counselling professions (Draft).* Lutterworth, UK: BACP.

Bentall, R. (2010). *Doctoring the mind: Why psychiatric treatments fail.* London: Penguin.

Bond, T. (2006). Intimacy, risk, and reciprocity in psychotherapy: Intricate ethical challenges. *Transactional Analysis Journal,* 36(2), 77–89.

Boston Change Process Study Group (2008). Forms of relational meaning: Issues in the relations between the implicit and reflective-verbal domains. *Psychoanalytic Dialogues,* 18, 125–48.

Foucault, M. (1977). *Discipline and punish: The birth of the prison.* Harmondsworth, UK: Penguin.

Garcia, R. (2008). *In treatment,* Series one. Los Angeles, CA: Home Box Office.

Gutheil, T. G. & Gabbard, G. O. (1993). The concept of boundaries in clinical practice: Theoretical and risk-management dimensions. *American Journal of Psychiatry,* 150, 189–96.

House, R. & Totton, N. (eds) (2011). *Implausible professions: Arguments for pluralism and autonomy in psychotherapy and counselling,* 2nd edn. Ross-on-Wye, UK: PCCS Books.

Lyon, D. (ed.) (2003). *Surveillance as social sorting: Privacy, risk, and digital discrimination.* London: Routledge.

Lyon, D. (2004). Surveillance technology and surveillance society. In J. M. Thomas, P. Brey, & A. Feenberg (eds), *Modernity and technology* (pp. 161–84). Cambridge, MA: MIT Press.

Malcolm, J. (2011). *Psychoanalysis: The impossible profession.* Cambridge, MA: Granta.

Maroda, K. (2002). *Seduction, surrender, and transformation: Emotional engagement in the analytic process.* Hove, UK: Psychology Press.

Mindell, A. (1985). *River's way: The process science of the dreambody.* London: Arkana.

Postle, D. (2007). *Regulating the psychological therapies: From taxonomy to taxidermy.* Ross-on-Wye, UK: PCCS Books.

Rose, N. & Abi-Rached, J. M. (2013). *Neuro: The new brain sciences and the management of the mind*. Princeton, NJ: Princeton University Press.

Totton, N. (2004). 'Can psychotherapy help make a better future?' Reprinted in N. Totton (2012), *Not a tame lion: Writings on therapy in its social and political context*. Ross-on-Wye, UK: PCCS Books, pp. 96–109.

Totton, N. (2008). 'In and out of the mainstream: Psychotherapy in its social and political contexts.' Reprinted in N. Totton (2012), *Not a tame lion: Writings on therapy in its social and political context*. Ross-on-Wye, UK: PCCS Books, pp. 115–27.

Totton, N. (2010). 'Boundaries and boundlessness.' Reprinted in N. Totton (2012), *Not a tame lion: Writings on therapy in its social and political context*. Ross-on-Wye, UK: PCCS Books, pp. 63–70.

Totton, N. (2011). *Wild therapy: Undomesticating inner and outer worlds*. Ross-on-Wye, UK: PCCS Books.

Totton, N. (2012). *Not a tame lion: Writings on therapy in its social and political context*. Ross-on-Wye, UK: PCCS Books.

11

BEYOND THE MEASURABLE

Alternatives to managed care in research and practice

Richard House

[T]he 'administrative and technological' have. . . penetrated the very lifeblood of our existence. . .

(van Manen, 1986, p. 29)

The client is not a 'dependent variable' to be operated on by an 'independent variable'.

(House & Bohart, 2008, p. 205)

Introduction

This chapter interrogates and critiques what can be termed 'the ideologies of modernity', exploring in the process some intrinsically unmeasurable phenomena that are argued to be central to the therapeutic experience – for example, subtlety, intuition, discernment, and 'the tacit' in human-relational experience. These crucial qualities rarely, if ever, figure in the kinds of empirical research that dominate our field, yet perversely, it is the overwhelmingly technical, manualised approaches that dominate managed-care and evidence-based driven therapy practice. If it is the case that *the spontaneous co-creation of human encounter* is one (if not *the*) core dimension to successful therapy practice, then manualised and related technical approaches are at best irrelevant and, at worst, actually detrimental to effective therapy practice. A kind of 'trance induction' has arguably been active in the case of the audit culture within therapy, with erstwhile critically minded practitioners seemingly taking the notion of 'evidence' and 'evidence-based practice', and the underlying dynamics driving these preoccupations, as unproblematic givens. In contrast, such modern totems of what I will call 'statist therapy' (i.e. IAPT, etc.) will be fundamentally problematised in what follows.

With the control-fixated 'manualisation' mentality that underpins 'statist therapy' fundamentally misrepresenting what actually happens in therapy practice by fetishising the conscious and the measurable, this chapter proposes an embodied, grounded approach to what is experienced in the therapy encounter, which accepts that not only can therapy outcome not be controlled or stipulated at the outset, but that the very act of trying so to do ends up throwing out the 'therapeutic baby', and so compromising and damaging the very essence of effective therapy.

Although strictly beyond the scope of this chapter, a full articulation of the argument would entail a full engagement with psycho-social critiques of the 'neo-liberal' paradigm and its associated mentality and discourses (e.g. Harvey, 2007; Peck, 2012), which currently hold such hegemonic and damaging sway in the hyper-audited National Health Service (House, 2012; Rizq, 2014), uncritically embedded as they are in the very psyches of managers and policy makers. From the perspective of therapy as a kind of (experiential) learning (Rose, Loewenthal, & Greenwood, 2005), the critical literature on pedagogy and neo-liberalism is certainly very relevant to these arguments (e.g. Hursh, 2006; de Lissovoy, 2013; Giroux, 2014; Hill, 2006), but will need to be pursued at another time.

Audit culture and the medical model

Modernity

A key assumption of this chapter is that it is essential to attempt to locate current developments in the therapy field within the wider evolution of human conscious-ness (e.g. Tarnas, 1991; Woodhouse, 1996; McGilchrist, 2012) – because only after such an attempt, no matter how inadequate or partial, will it be possible to understand at all comprehensively just what is driving what we might call a kind of paradigm-bound 'acting-out' in the policy-making arena. On this view, therapy 'needs to be critically and reflexively located within its evolving historical, cultural and paradigmatic context' (House, Karian, & Young, 2011, p. 180) (cf. Levin, 1987; Cushman, 1995).

In McGilchrist's terms, for example, within state-defined 'therapy' (with the quote marks denoting whether it is even legitimate to consider such practices to be authentic therapy at all, in any meaningful sense), we are currently living through an era in which an inferior, control-fixated, instrumental-mechanistic 'left-brain' mentality is dominating modern Western culture, with (in McGilchrist's view) catastrophic consequences for the ways in which we live our lives and understand our world. Not that these arguments are especially new, for back in the early to mid-1990s, Gill Edwards (1992) was asking whether psychotherapy needs 'a soul'; in the same year, Ann Schaef was proposing a paradigm for therapy that moves beyond the constraining mentality of modernity (Shaef, 1992; see also House, 2003); and the current author was challenging the rise of 'audit-mindedness' in GP counselling (House, 1996; see also King & Moutsou, 2010). Part of this telling psycho-social story is the key role that *unprocessed anxiety* plays in social formations and in the policy-making process, right down to the detail of policy-making itself (Cooper, 2001; Fotaki, 2006). More on this later.

Audit-culture managerialism

> Audit culture is a product of this drive toward marketization, but it is also itself an important vehicle for marketization and commodification.
>
> *(Thorpe, 2008, p. 105)*

What, after James Nolan, we might call the 'therapeutic state' (Nolan, 1998) is being increasingly fashioned in the image of the neo-liberal capitalist economy, and the economic imperatives and ideological practices that accompany it. This in turn will tend to generate what post-modern theorist David Harvey (1973) has called 'status-quo theory' – that is, theory, research and professional practice which merely serve to reinforce the distributional, structural and materialist status quo, rather than generating knowledge and practice that can help us to transcend the limitations of the status quo. An in-built bias towards status quo conservatism is thus almost inevitable in a regulatory system which pre-decides 'standards' and 'competencies' which must then be followed or met.

As early as the 1980s, the recently deceased psychologist David Smail was also prophetically insightful into the inherently conservative, even reactionary, function that 'therapy' could serve in the wrong hands (e.g. Smail, 1983, 1987, 1996). Nearly 30 years ago, for example, he wrote: 'through becoming unthinkingly over-extended, [psychotherapy] is in danger of being ethically misused or abused. In order to guard against such misuse, psychotherapists must beware of slipping into the role of established and technically sound professional expert' (Smail, 1987, p. 43) – which is, of course, precisely the role played by the new state-therapy 'regime of truth' into which compliant practitioners are now being forced. Certainly, Smail argued forcefully that it is precisely the kinds of values and ideologies that lie at the heart of the audit culture's bludgeon that have so often damaged the clients who look for help and support for that damage when they seek out therapeutic help.

Just how authentic is any help that therapists offer to such clients when those practitioners have colluded with pernicious cultural forces, which it should surely be the place of critically minded psycho-cultural commentators and therapists fearlessly to deconstruct and challenge? What I will term 'authentic therapy practice' (as distinct from 'state therapy') can only be conducted by practitioners who explicitly and self-reflexively undertake to strive for a deep congruence between their face-to-face work with clients, on the one hand and, on the other, the approach they take to, and the relationship they have with, the prevailing cultural *Zeitgeist* and all its psycho-social machinations and vicissitudes.

Instrumental thinking (Foucault and Heidegger), the ubiquitous 'audit culture' (see Power, 1997) with its catastrophic impact upon public services and education, and the imperatives of global capital accumulation which 'annihilates space by time'

(Marx, cited in Noys, 2014) together constitute a noxious combination of forces and influences that cannot but severely compromise, if not almost eradicate, the free counter-cultural space in which the erstwhile unthinkable can begin to be thought, and which genuine therapy, at its best, stands for. Such a free space is an essential prerequisite for the kind of genuine change that therapy promises, unconstrained by familial and cultural regimes of truth that can only generate compliance rather than authentic change.

Concern about the so-called 'audit culture' has received growing attention since the 1990s, and has now even reached the psychotherapy literature itself (most notably, see Power, 1998; Cooper, 2001; King & Moutsou, 2010). As newspaper editor Peter Preston once wrote, 'We now live in a relentlessly superintended world, a quangoed regime of commissioners, inspectors, and regulators. . . . Fundamental principles about freedom, autonomy, and citizenship are threatened by this state of affairs. . . . Obsessional activity . . . is essentially about control rather than creativity' (cited in Cooper, 2001, *passim*). And if 'standards' *are* to be a legitimate concern, then more disturbingly still, such systems may well be contributing to a *deterioration* of standards, while maintaining the pretence that they are achieving the opposite (ibid.).

While one might charitably presume that the conscious intention of apologists for the audit and accountability culture in state therapy is that of improving the effectiveness of the therapy experience, quite other (neo-liberal, paradigm-bound) agendas are likely operating at individual and collective-unconscious levels.

There exists an incommensurability between, on the one hand, the state's drive for standardisation and common, universal standards of service provision in state therapy and, on the other, flexible responsiveness to the particularities and uniqueness of clients' experience (cf. Bohart & House, 2008). Critical, independent thinking is one of the first casualties of any mind-set that expediently embraces the principle of generic standardisation and the alleged, but chimerical, virtues of state regulation of a field as diverse as ours. These developments also represent a critical shift in the locus of power away from the professional autonomy of practitioners themselves, and towards managerialist imperatives and administrative bureaucratic interests (a story that can no doubt be re-told many times throughout the public services; Parker, 2002). And of key importance is that the axioms of the audit-driven paradigm will routinely influence, or even *construct*, the very ways in which practitioners and professionals conceive of, and think about, their work and their very professional identities within such regimes of truth.

Such an audit-driven, calculation-obsessed worldview is arguably quite unable to embrace ambiguity, not-knowing, the intuitive and the mysterious (Cayne & Loewenthal, 2008); and so one of the first casualties of this ideology will be any approach to therapy that sees as central the embracing of ambiguity and dialectical thinking in its practice, and which does not conform to any linear, predictable and controllable process or monolithic logic.

There is no doubt a telling, if complex and overdetermined psychoanalytic story to be told about the audit culture, and the economic, cultural and individual dynamics underpinning and driving it (for some useful beginnings, see Cooper, 2001; Miller, 2007; Rizq, 2014). Such crucial engagements, and the theoretical labour they require, lie beyond the scope and intention of this chapter. But theoretical insight also needs to be balanced with a committed praxis, engaging fully with the particular political and strategic challenges to which audit culture mentalities and practices give rise in our daily lives.

There are a number of interrelated reasons why the audit culture perpetrates such damage to human services in which *relational* considerations, qualities and sensibilities are paramount. First, in a short-term kind of political system, Government targets will tend to be manipulatively and expediently politicised. A targeting fixation is also intrinsically distorting, not merely because quantitative indicators can never capture the complexities and subtleties of therapy experience, but because *the indicators themselves* become more important than the qualities they are purported to measure (particularly when punitive 'name and shame' is the threatened result of 'statistical failure') – with public service workers and politicians alike focusing all their energies on meeting the crude targets, while the far more subtle and complex issues of true quality are ignored.

Distortions are then further exacerbated when those subjected to this low-trust 'surveillance culture' can 'cook' the indicators not by *genuine* improvements, but by wasting resources outmanoeuvring the assessment system. Next, the very mentality which has been imposed upon the system in order to 'deliver' the targets (narrow, utilitarian etc.) will tend systematically to have compromised and denuded much that was of real value in the pre-targeting era. Finally, the testing and/or targeting regime – as with all technocratic intrusions into human systems – leads to quite unpredictable side-effects which commonly do more net harm than do the improvements they are supposed to effect. A clear example in 'state therapy' would be where an agenda of getting 'patients' back into the workforce can easily serve to distract therapists and patients from engaging with the therapeutic work that the patients need for their own healing.

The so-called 'managerialism' (Parker, 2002) also goes hand in hand with the audit culture. Thus, there is a common tendency under neo-liberalism to define social, economic and political issues as problems that can best be resolved through management, and with managerialism or the New Public Management constituting a new mode of governance in Western countries' restructured public sectors (e.g. Diefenbach, 2009). Tellingly, such managerialism draws theoretically on *corporate* and private sector management styles, and also on public choice theory and new institutional economics (e.g. agency theory and transaction cost analysis).

In the New Public Management or the New Managerialism, with their 'rationalised performance criteria', knowledge is 'commodified so as to make it a useful product of pre-ordained and pre-conceived . . . directives and scientific outcomes not necessarily for the sake of science, truth or knowledge' (Trifonas, 2004, p. 39). Far from supporting and encouraging a free climate of relatively unconstrained creativity and learning that therapy at its best requires, such a regime has the effect of reversing the conditions under which an innovative milieu flourishes.

The therapeutic space cast in the image of neo-liberal late modernity is therefore moving away from its formerly more open counter-cultural nature where the previously 'unthought' has a space in which to emerge, with even more infiltration of 'neo-liberal' driven, control-oriented State influence, and a stultifying and anxiety-inculcating culture of surveillance, audit and bureaucratic control. What we are witnessing, in short, is an economy-driven neo-liberal, even quasi-authoritarian colonisation of the therapy experience.

At a psychosocial level, more generally, it can also be argued that modern Western culture is teetering under the weight of unprecedented levels of unacknowledged and unprocessed anxiety, which in turn is toxically infecting our public institutions, including the state's annexation of therapy. As a result, it can be argued that policy-makers are in some sense 'acting out' in all manner of highly dysfunctional and inappropriate ways, in the process exposing our clients to the full force of a soullessly utilitarian regime that has little to do with clients' genuine therapeutic needs, and everything to do with the *Zeitgeist* of Late Modernity, the hyper-competitive globalised economy, and even policy makers' 'learned helplessness' in the face of these global forces.

So what is to be done, as the 'politicization' of therapy becomes a cultural norm in Late Modernity, and without any seriously informed public debate? The psycho(social) dynamics that are underpinning and driving these cultural developments need to be fully theorised and articulated – a task, surely, for critically minded therapists and psychosocial commentators to engage with.

'State therapy' in the audit culture

Many, if not most, therapists are very critical of the inappropriateness of 'shoe-horning' what is at core a non-positivistic, post-modern healing practice into an alien audit culture, standardising an ideology whose assumptions do a kind of violence to the nature of our work. Standardisation-obsessed policy-makers seem either quite unable to grasp, or else are determined wilfully to ignore, the subtleties and nuances of the activity of therapy.

With the ideology of standardisation being rooted in a normalising, Late-Modernist worldview that, for many, if not the majority, of therapists, fundamentally misunderstands, misrepresents and even does a kind of violence to core therapy values, which at their best are striving to transcend the crude bludgeon of Late Modernity, in what direction is state therapy currently taking us? First, medical-model developments in the 'psy' field (Skills for Health, IAPT etc.) will tend to reduce access to long-term, relationally oriented therapy and counselling; reduce client choice; medicalise the field; and rigidify training and inflate its cost and hence the cost of therapy, making access to appropriate therapy help even more difficult for the economically disadvantaged and the minorities.

Counselling and psychotherapy are inherently 'risky': they cannot be made to conform to a 'safety-first' culture, and any attempt to do so can only degrade the quality of help offered, and encourage a limited kind of 'defensive psychotherapy'. As Mowbray (1995, p. 150) writes,

> What is fostered by such circumstances is not a fertile and innovative field
> but conformity of practice based not so much on true standards . . . as on
> practitioner self-protection – the practice of 'defensive psychotherapy'.
> Practitioners will do or not do things in order to avoid disciplinary action,
> malpractice suits and/or the invalidating of their insurance cover, rather than
> solely on the basis of whether or not the client would benefit.

At worst, we will likely end up with a programmatic kind of therapy that becomes
little more than an apology for the cultural status quo (cf. Harvey, 1973). For the
delicate field of therapy work is one of the last places where managerialist, 'audit
culture' values and practices should hold sway. A 'standardisation ideology' saturated
the worldview underpinning the previous government's intention to state-regulate
the psychological therapies. Their White Paper, 'Trust, Assurance and Safety – The
Regulation of Health Professionals in the Twenty-first Century' (Secretary of State
for Health, February 2007, Cm 7013), was shot through with the ideology of
standardisation – and all the associated violence that such a mentality threatens to
perpetrate on the rich diversity of therapy practice. For example, on page 85, para
7.17 of the White Paper, we read the following extraordinary assertion: the
Government believes that all professionals undertaking the same activity should be
subject to the same standards of training and practice so that those who use their
services can be assured that there is no difference in quality'. This single sentence
grafts so many misunderstandings upon multiple misunderstandings about therapy
practice that it is difficult to know where to begin.

Back in 1997, the Senior Policy Advisor on regulation in the Department of
Health, Anne Richardson, acknowledged publicly that psychotherapy was a hugely
diverse 'activity' (her term; cited in House & Totton, 2011b, p. 10), so to refer
to 'the same activity' in this context is essentially meaningless; the phrase 'the same
standards of . . . practice' is again to misunderstand an activity that is intrinsically
unauditable and uncontrollable through the kind of 'managerialist' definitional fiat
beloved of the Health and Care Professions Council; and finally, the very idea that
it is appropriate and possible that clients be 'assured' that there is no difference in
quality between practitioners' 'services' represents a wholly inappropriate intrusion
of normalising consumerist values into therapy work.

'State therapy' assumes that counselling and psychotherapy constitute activities
for which it is possible in principle, and appropriate in practice, to define
universalising generic standards, that can be generalised across the psy field. But
this is fundamentally a misunderstanding of the unique and subtle nature of therapy
practice, uncritically embracing, as it does, a Late-Modernist paradigm (including
the anxiety-driven surveillance and audit cultures) just at the time when, culturally
and historically, the paradigm of 'modernity' is under sustained philosophical,
political and spiritual challenge in a whole host of ways. The psychological therapies
should surely be at the forefront of these paradigmatic challenges, and should
certainly not be colluding with and reinforcing a moribund paradigm of Late
Modernity in its death throes (Barratt, 1993).

The issue of incommensurable paradigms (in the Kuhnian sense) becomes most acute here; for from a 'new paradigm', transpersonal or trans-critical post-modern perspective – which privileges, for example, the unknown, unlearning, 'negative capability' (Keats) and practising 'without memory or desire' (Bion) – the specification of standards and competencies 'before the event' is fundamentally to misunderstand and to misspecify that which is central in the practice of many therapists in their work.

Lynn Fendler (1998, p. 57), for example, has developed the kind of critique of the standards-obsessed positivistic discourse that has been notably missing in any deliberations about the appropriateness of state-regulating psy activity via a standards-based ideology. Below, I reproduce an aspect of her incisive critique, substituting 'therapy' for 'education' terms (as exactly the same arguments apply in both fields):

> Now there is a reversal; the goals and outcomes are being stipulated at the outset, and the procedures are being developed post hoc. The 'nature' of the [client's experience] is stipulated in advance, based on objective criteria, usually statistical analysis. Because the outcome drives the procedure (rather than vice versa), there is no longer the theoretical possibility of unexpected results; there is no longer the theoretical possibility of becoming unique in the process of becoming ['treated'] . . . In this new system, evaluation of [psychotherapeutic] policy reform is limited to an evaluation of the degree to which any given procedure yields the predetermined results.

There surely exist very considerable dangers indeed in the therapy world engaging with this pernicious *Zeitgeist* – one which is arguably quite antithetical to the core values of therapeutic work at its best, and of which standards-driven 'state therapy' can be seen to be the crowning 'glory'. One reason why therapy has arguably been such an effective and successful cultural practice over many decades is precisely because there has not (yet) been any concerted attempt to control, 'can' and colonise 'therapy' in relation to any external or 'statist' agenda to which therapy has increasingly become subject in recent years.

This view is also entirely consistent with Rudolf Steiner's conception of the Threefold Social Order (lying, crucially, beyond both socialism and capitalism) (Steiner, 1919/1996; see also Large, 2010), in which it is seen as essential that the activity of the cultural sphere in society is left relatively free from, and unhindered by, either political (politicised) or financial/economic interests.

Historically, counselling and psychotherapy have been conducted in a private, confidential space, free of externally defined, institutionally driven agendas, in which clients can take matters of deep personal concern for dialogical exploration and reflection. The therapeutic space is arguably one of Late-Modern society's last surviving refuges from narrowly stultifying mechanistic thinking, and from the intrusive compliance experiences that bring many, if not most, clients into therapy in the first place (cf. Smail, 1987).

The State's intrusion into what should be a culturally unique private space, with its control-fixated agenda which is only capable of 'seeing like a State' (Nolan, 1998), can only compromise the quality of that space. There is an urgent need to protect the therapy space from this unwarranted government colonisation; and recent developments can only fuel suspicions that the State's annexation of therapy for its own ends is merely the latest symptom of a wider cultural movement towards a 'surveillance society', in which, not least, therapy becomes inappropriately annexed to a governmental social-engineering agenda. For some years now, Totton (e.g. 2011, p. 3) has argued that '[W]e made a very bad decision when we chose to bring therapy within the NHS', and it seems that he is proving to be right (for a fuller, critical discussion of this debate, see House, 2012).

'Intangibles' and the 'post-modern turn' in therapy

> Therapy 'works' through the interrelational *presence* of the therapist, rather than through specific technological or skill-based operations.
>
> *(Bohart & House, 2008, p. 195)*

'Post-modernism' is not an 'ism', or any kind of thing, but rather, a key transitional moment in the evolution of ideas and human consciousness – a moment denoting both an important disillusionment with the objectivist Enlightenment project of modernity, and a liminal potential space which presages something that is as yet unknown and undefined (and may, of course, remain intrinsically so, as 'knowing' and 'definition' themselves are increasingly problematised). Over several decades, there has been a 'post-modern turn' in psychoanalysis, psychotherapy and psychology (e.g. Faulconer & Williams, 1990; Kvale, 1992; Barratt, 1993; Anderson, 1997; Parker, 1999; Frie, 2003; House, 2003), prompted by a profound epistemological and political disillusionment with the therapy profession's perceived capture by the ideology of modernity, with its accompanying belief in

- a referential-representational view of language;
- individual autonomy and rationality on the part of analysts/therapists or patients/clients (knowers and the known);
- historical, scientific and disciplinary progress;
- the desirability of grand and unifying theories and singular forms of knowing; and
- objective and disinterested knowledge and professional expertise (Lowe, 1999, p. 75).

In general terms, the 'post-modern' signifies ways of perceiving, experiencing and behaving which relax and challenge the taken-for-granted assumptions that dominate the Cartesian Enlightenment thinking of 'modernity' in the West. In recent decades, many of these assumptions have come under searching critique from manifold sources.

But what does or could such a 'post-modern' therapy look like in practice? Stemming from a conference workshop on accountability in the psy therapies in 2011, House *et al.* (2011, p. 180) drew up the following list of core values of therapy work:

- therapy is most accurately characterised as a hermeneutic, meaning-discovering and/or meaning-creating process, making it far more akin to a relational art than a science;
- therapy privileges 'the emergent' in the work – i.e. ethical therapeutic practice cannot be protocol driven, and so does not specify *at the outset* what the goals, targets or outcomes of therapy are or should be: rather, an 'opening-up' space is created such that a client's issues of concern can emerge, with the therapist being non-judgementally open to whatever issues the client might wish to bring;
- the change process within therapy is intrinsically unpredictable and uncontrollable via the kinds of 'modernist' control agendas that typify therapy when conceived as a medical-model, remedial 'technology';
- therapy at its pluralistic best strives to transcend modality sectarianism, and to privilege a non-defended openness and flexibility when working with the emergent;
- therapy is non-utilitarian, in that it does not *necessarily* entail any wish to maximize 'happiness' or 'well-being' (e.g. Woolfolk, 2002; Pilgrim, 2008; van Deurzen, 2009); and
- therapy practice should be *values based* rather than evidence based (McCarthy & Rose, 2010), such that the totems of positivistic science are not uncritically privileged over values and ethics (e.g. Gantt, 2000).

It should be clear from this list that these values and principles (to which I suspect the vast majority of therapists would willingly and enthusiastically subscribe) is a million miles away from the kind of state-delivered 'therapy' which I am fundamentally problematising in this chapter.

In Bohart and House (2008) and House and Bohart (2008), the authors have set out at great length just what the differences are, epistemologically and ontologically, between the kind of 'state therapy' which I am challenging in this chapter, and the kind of 'post-modern' therapy which is far more consistent with the core values of psychotherapy (listed above). I will summarise some of the key arguments here.

For the philosopher of science, Kuhn (1977), it is generally difficult for those speaking from different paradigms or 'world-views' to understand one another, not least because of the incommensurable and often unarticulated assumptions from which each speaks, and it seems that this may be at least part of the problem in the way in which statist therapy and what I call authentic, 'post-modern' therapy miss one another. The proponents of statist therapy commonly fail to recognise the paradigmatic or ontological level from which objections to its approach are being raised, and some of which I mention in this chapter.

From a more post-modern perspective, for example, it is unwise prematurely to impose a unitary, standardising paradigm on to a field, when that paradigm has not been consensually arrived at and ignores a whole historical tradition of effective therapeutic work, and has been managerialistically created by a minority of people in a narrowly circumscribed part of the field. On this view, then, attempts to entrench 'statist therapy' assumptions as *the* (only) route to legitimate practice constitutes a hegemonic attempt to impose on both science and practice what is to us, at least in part, an alien and epistemologically unsustainable world-view.

The 'paradigm war' in therapy, then, is being fought out between a 'modernist', Newtonian view of the universe, with its goal of increasing control over dependent variables by specifying and manipulating independent variables, and a more holistic 'post-modern' cosmology, where we can never totally predict or control the phenomena being studied, and where 'science' is acknowledged, but without it necessarily determining or dominating practice. Post-modern cosmology also actively welcomes and celebrates a rich diversity of alternative therapy paradigms (House & Totton, 2011); yet CBT and statist therapy, as modernity's paradigm-crowning modality (House & Loewenthal, 2008), are severely limiting the therapy that is available through the State and the NHS to a narrowly circumscribed, instrumental 'technology' of therapy that bears little if any relation to the kind of authentic, post-modern therapy that I am advocating in this chapter.

In its underlying logic, the statist-therapy paradigm makes major assumptions concerning the nature of psychotherapy, underpinned in turn by a more general metaphysical position which necessarily entails implicit and interconnected assumptions about reality, science, knowledge and truth. Thus, in this paradigm, psychotherapy practice is viewed through an analogy to the medical model, with a central focus upon treatment, which is viewed as analogous to drug treatment, and which seeks to 'correct' abnormal, so-called 'psychopathology' (Parker, Georgaca, Harper & McLaughlin, 1995), just as drugs are supposed to correct or cure 'pathology'. On this modernist view, it is believed that the treatment qua treatment is somehow applied to the problem or 'disorder' in a causal way, so as to eradicate it. Within this world-view, therapy becomes a technological enterprise, with, at worst, 'therapists viewed as "behavioral engineers" rather than storytellers or moral guides' (Johnson & Sandage, 1999, p. 4).

The 'treatment', then, is effectively the independent variable, which is applied to the 'dependent variable' – the client (or the client's 'disorder'), the goal being to 'operationalise' the treatment clearly and unambiguously. The more precisely the independent variable can be operationalised, the better for plotting predictable linear-causal relationships between it and the dependent variable. Within this paradigm, 'ill-defined' or 'non-specific' common factors, such as 'the relationship' dimension and other unmeasurable human qualities, cannot be specified or operationalised as a series of unambiguously definable, measurable and controllable therapist strategies, and so are left out of account.

Yet if, as many practitioners believe, it is precisely these difficult-to-define 'imponderables' that are most important in many a healing and change experience (see below), then to embrace an approach which systematically rules them out of account, and which privileges, instead, only that which is measurable and controllable, may well be to do a kind of procedural violence to therapeutic reality as widely understood in the field.

In the authentic post-modern paradigm, by contrast, the therapist as person is working with a whole person in order to help the latter remove obstacles to living what, for them, is a more fulfilling life, with the therapist relying upon the clients' own capacities for self-healing (Bohart & Tallman, 1996). The client's own 'generativity' is an integral part of this process, and insights and solutions emerge from therapist and client interrelating, rather than being dictated a priori by a 'cookbook' list of treatments matched up to problems, conditions or diagnoses.

In contrast to the idea that the therapist is 'treating' a 'disorder', then, therapy becomes a co-created dialogue between two (or more) intelligent, living, embodied beings. The guiding metaphor for this approach is therefore conversation and healing dialogue (e.g. Anderson, 1997), and therapy is no more seen as a medical-like treatment. And it is the 'being' of the therapist and client in indissoluble relationship which is assumed to be therapeutic, and not specific 'therapist operations', skills or programmatic interventions. And the therapist works with moment-to-moment phenomenological sensitivity to the subtlety and complexity of the emerging process, depending upon their ability to respond appropriately in that moment. This kind of view is very difficult to understand from a modernist paradigmatic position, which claims that only what is definable and measurable has meaning and effectivity – or even can be said to exist! There may be, and probably is, a potentially infinite set of different ways in which therapists could embody and actualise the relational qualities of warmth, empathy and genuineness with different clients. It therefore seems particularly absurd to think of many therapists all trying to 'provide' the same 'intervention' in a standardised fashion, when what is so clearly healing about a given unique contextual experience is arguably its natural spontaneity and human quality.

The paradigm alternative to statist therapy that I am describing here has subtlety, intuition, the tacit, spontaneity and a 'uniqueness assumption' at its core, with psychotherapy conceived of as a practice which has the idiographic aim of focusing on the unique, particular individual case or situation. Effective and successful practitioners treat each new client (and session) as unique; for as DeGreene has it, 'The concept of clearly definable and correlatable independent, intervening and dependent variables may be completely inappropriate in a dynamic, mutually causal world' (DeGreene, 1991, as quoted in Nadler, Hibino & Farrell, 1995, p. 89). The uniqueness assumption therefore means that the practitioner focuses on the particulars of each individual case, rather than on how a given case fits into a general category (Schön, 1983).

In the authentic-therapy paradigm, the two complex intersubjective 'systems', namely, the therapist and client, influence one another and psychically interpenetrate in a multitude of different and often unspecifiable ways: verbally, non-verbally, emotionally, cognitively, perceptually, behaviourally, and even spiritually or transpersonally. These multiple paths of influence cross and re-cross in dynamic, circular, non-linearly causal ways; and so a 'meeting of persons' is a complex, indissolubly holistic phenomenon which simply cannot be dismantled into component, linear causal parts.

Moreover, in this cosmology, therapeutic interventions simply do not map in a one-to-one fashion into client effects, but rather set up perturbations in complex ecological systems where, at best, all we will ever be able to expect are partial, incomplete, and therefore quite possibly misleading correlations between inputs and ultimate outputs. And effective practitioners learn how to use their intuition to transcend rules, progressively acquiring a much more subtle and differentiated tacit knowledge of the terrain of practice than can ever, in principle, be expressed in explicit rules or protocols. In this paradigm, then, a starting assumption is that each practitioner–client pair will generate its own unique ways of working effectively. Different practitioners will embody practice principles in different ways; and in all cases of practice, the role of the practitioner is crucial.

Rather than setting out manipulatively to control the world (as the technocratic objectivist does), the sensitive practitioner offers the possibility of in-touch contact with, and full participation in, the 'life-world', privileging sensitivity, openness to existential experience, and a commitment to inquire into lived, revealed meaning. Key reference texts for the authentic paradigm are Schön (1983) and Atkinson and Claxton (2000).

For Atkinson and Claxton, intuition plays a crucial role in the exercising and development of professional decision-making and judgement. The 'modernist' tendency to 'fetishise' the conscious and the declarative, and to interpret reflection solely in terms of conscious articulation, is fundamentally questioned, and the value of forms of reflection that are not necessarily articulatable is strongly asserted.

If it is true that qualities like subtlety, discernment, and intuitive capacity are key common-factor 'ingredients' of effective practitionership, and if those very qualities are not only not amenable to the positivistic 'violence' that is 'variable specification' and all that goes with it, but are actually adversely affected by such an 'evidence-based' mentality, then it may well be that the very act of importing a 'politically correct' preoccupation with accountability into our work substantially compromises it. It even ends up with the grotesque outcome that our anxiety-driven need to somehow guarantee the efficacy of our work, and the armamentarium of procedures that we adopt to prove it, actually do far more net damage to the quality of therapy work than any improvements brought about by the assessment and accountability regime itself.

Crassly positivistic and technocratic conceptions of service evaluation – what Kilroy, Bailey and Chare (2004, p. 1) refer to as 'the reduction of (qualitative) thought to (quantitative) product, (critical) education to (utilitarian) skill-set' – are surely singularly inappropriate means of evaluating efficacy in the peculiarly unique and idiosyncratic field of psychotherapeutic help. For as Broadfoot has it, 'attempts to pretend that a human being's achievements, or even more, their potential, can be unambiguously measured, are doomed from the outset' (2000, p. 215).

What our field should surely be embracing is the most radical thinking in relevant and associated fields (e.g. Trifonas, 2004), rather than uncritically mimicking the worst features of the 'surveillance culture' and the soulless technocracies of 'high modernity'.

Implications for a grounded approach to therapy

In a world of 'post-modernity' that fundamentally questions the ideologies of (hyper-)modernity that this chapter squarely rejects, I would argue that the kind of counselling work which I and many of my colleagues did within General Practice in the NHS between 1990 and 2007 (House, 2004) could be a model for the kind of 'non-statist', nascent post-modern therapy I wish to advocate here.

In my own practice as a GP counsellor between 1990 and 2006, I have found it eminently possible to work in a very creative and responsive way with clients – especially as the majority of clients came into GP counselling without any preconceptions about therapy and the 'rules' of how to be a good therapy client; and, as a result, they often entered into a cocreative dialogic relationship with enthusiasm, ease and a minimum of mystification – a meeting which naturally seemed to embrace many if not most of the characteristics of a post-modern approach to therapy listed earlier (House *et al.*, 2011).

A case in point is the phenomenon of *flexibility*. Lees (1997) advocates a Winnicottian-style flexibility for the GP therapeutic framework in which the practitioner is exquisitely sensitive and responsive to the dialectical 'dance' between flexibility and firmness – rather than pre-emptively assuming that firm, 'holding' boundaries are essential.

In addition, it is precisely because the GP setting is a medical setting that it offers an excellent opportunity for practitioners (if unconstrained by statist protocols) to explore ways of *transcending* simplistic mind/body dualism, and of working holistically and creatively with so-called 'psychosomatic' symptoms. My strong hunch is that back in the 1990s, there was a significant amount of highly innovative, path-breaking therapeutic work being done in GP settings in Britain, and that such innovations would, in time, have diffused into the therapy field more generally in quite unforeseeable ways, if the CBT and IAPT juggernaut hadn't virtually extinguished this pioneering work virtually overnight in the mid to late 2000s.

Conclusion: therapy in a high-trust world

> Perhaps the moment will come when we will burn the questionnaires . . . and when we will refuse to print the questionnaires with their little boxes, because those little boxes we tick will be the death of us.
>
> *(Miller, 2007, p. 28)*

A central assumption of this chapter is that *not* to attempt to locate therapeutic practices and their assumptive philosophies within the evolution of ideas and human consciousness is a major (and telling) omission, and I have tried to do this in this chapter in relation to the sharply incommensurable paradigms of 'statist' and authentic, post-modern therapy. The managerial world of audit, accountability and 'evidence-based practice' (Trinder & Reynolds, 2000; Mace, Moorey & Roberts, 2001) is typified by the need to control and make safe, driven by unprocessed anxiety and an associated low-trust mentality, and a neo-liberal ideology, such that such practices are inherently conservative, unimaginative and reinforcing of the status quo. I maintain that at this juncture the State is only able to see in certain ways (Scott, 1999), and this means that statist therapy is necessarily limited, constraining and only able to reinforce the status quo rather than being a crucible for transcending it. So there is arguably some kind of insidious process operating in modern culture such that we can all end up 'thinking like a state' (Scott, 1999) – with all of the deadly, limiting and distorting consequences of that surreptitious mentality. Broadfoot puts it thus:

> assessment is . . . so central to the discourse of contemporary culture that [quoting Wittgenstein] we find ourselves in a 'linguistic prison'; we have been 'bewitched' by the concepts of . . . assessment . . . to such an extent that even what we are able to think is constrained by the boundaries of that conceptual language.
>
> *(2000, p. 207)*

In other words, the 'audit culture' and its accompanying ideology are systematically saturating every aspect of public and, increasingly, private life, and therapy is by no means immune from these arguably toxic developments.

Miller (2002) has written an engaging book on 'postmodern public policy', in which he maintains that 'rationality has over-extended its capacity to rationalise and is beginning to undo itself' (p. x), and arguing further for a new 'bottom-up policy discourse' that challenges technical-instrumental thought, and which seems to me to sit very well with the kind of authentic post-modern paradigm championed here. For as Shaef put it over 20 years ago:

> Psychotherapists . . . must make a paradigm shift . . . [They] can recover from their enmeshment in a paradigm that does not work for us, and as we do, our work will be completely different. . . . It is not possible to use the techniques and philosophies of the mechanistic paradigm to heal the effects and devastations of that paradigm.
>
> *(Schaef, 1992, p. 307)*

I submit, in closing, that therapists now have a clear choice: we can either comply and collude with the forces of Late Modernity and neo-liberalism colonising the consulting room, or we can stay true to therapy's proud counter-cultural and paradigm-transcending roots, and say a firm 'No' to the alien forces of statist therapy that have been foisted upon us in recent years. And the future of our work, and its very nature, depend on the choice we will make, individually and collectively. It is morally incumbent on us all to make the right one.

References

Anderson, H. (1997). *Conversation, language, and possibilities: A postmodern approach to therapy.* New York: Basic Books.

Atkinson, T. & Claxton, G. (eds) (2000). *The intuitive practitioner: On the value of not always knowing what one is doing.* Buckingham, UK: Open University Press.

Barratt, B. B. (1993). *Psychoanalysis and the postmodern impulse: Knowing and being since Freud's psychology.* Baltimore, MD: Johns Hopkins University Press.

Bohart, A. C. & House, R. (2008). Empirically supported/validated treatments as modernist ideology, I: Dodo, manualization, and the paradigm question. In R. House & D. Loewenthal (eds), *Against and for CBT: Towards a constructive dialogue?* (pp. 188–201). Ross-on-Wye, UK: PCCS Books.

Bohart, A. C. & Tallman, K. A. (1996). The active client: Therapy as self-help. *Journal of Humanistic Psychology*, 36(3), 7–30.

Broadfoot, P. (2000). Assessment and intuition. In T. Atkinson & G. Claxton (eds), *The intuitive practitioner: On the value of not always knowing what one is doing* (pp. 199–219). Buckingham, UK: Open University Press.

Cayne, J. & Loewenthal, D. (2008). The between as unknown. *Philosophical Practice*, 3(3), 322–32.

Cooper, A. (2001). The state of mind we're in: Social anxiety, governance and the audit society. *Psychoanalytic Studies*, 3(3–4), 349–62.

Cushman, P. (1995). *Constructing the self, constructing America: A cultural history of psychotherapy.* Reading, MA: Addison-Wesley.

de Lissovoy, N. (2013). Pedagogy of the impossible: Neoliberalism and the ideology of accountability. *Policy Futures in Education*, 11(4). Available at: www.wwwords.co.uk/rss/abstract.asp?j=pfie&aid=5570.

DeGreene, K. B. (1991). Rigidity and fragility of large sociotechnical systems: Advanced information technology, the dominant coalition, and paradigm shift at the end of the twentieth century. *Behavioral Science*, 36, 64–79.

Diefenbach, T. (2009). New public management in public sector organizations: The dark sides of managerialistic 'enlightenment'. *Public Administration*, 87(4), 892–909.

Edwards, G. (1992). Does psychotherapy need a soul? In W. Dryden & C. Feltham (eds), *Psychotherapy and its discontents* (pp. 194–224). Buckingham, UK: Open University Press.

Faulconer, J. E. & Williams, R. N. (eds) (1990). *Reconsidering psychology: Perspectives from continental philosophy.* Pittsburgh, PA: Duquesne University Press.

Fendler, L. (1998). What is it impossible to think? A genealogy of the educated subject. In T. S. Popkewitz & M. Brennan (eds), *Foucault's challenge: Discourse, knowledge and power in education* (pp. 39–63). New York: Teachers College Press, Columbia University.

Fotaki, M. (2006). Choice is yours: A psychodynamic exploration of health policymaking and its consequences for the English National Health Service. *Human Relations*, 59(12), 1711–1744.

Frie, R. (ed.). (2003). *Understanding experience: Psychotherapy and postmodernism.* London: Routledge.

Gantt, E. E. (2000). Levinas, psychotherapy, and the ethics of suffering. *Journal of Humanistic Psychology*, 40(3), 9–28.

Giroux, H. A. (2014). *Higher education after neoliberalism.* Chicago, IL: Haymarket Books.

Harvey, D. (1973). *Social justice and the city*. London: Edward Arnold (revised edn, 2009).

Harvey, D. (2007). *A brief history of neoliberalism*. Oxford: Oxford University Press.

Hill, D. (2006). Educational perversion and global neoliberalism. In E. W. Ross and R. Gibson (eds), Neoliberalism and education reform (pp. 107–44). Cresskill, NJ: Hampton Press.

Hill, D. (2007). *Neoliberalism and the perversion of education*. In E. W. Ross & R. Gibson (eds), *Neoliberalism and education reform*. Cresskill, NJ: Hampton Press.

House, R. (1996). 'Audit-mindedness' in counselling: Some underlying dynamics. *British Journal of Guidance and Counselling*, 24(2), 277–83. Reprinted in R. House and N. Totton (eds), *Implausible professions: Arguments for pluralism and autonomy in psychotherapy and counselling*, 2nd edn (pp. 74–82). Ross-on Wye, UK: PCCS Books.

House, R. (2003). *Therapy beyond modernity: Deconstructing and transcending profession-centred therapy*. London: Karnac Books.

House, R. (2004). General practice counselling: Nascent postmodern therapy? *Psychodynamic Practice*, 10(3), 394–99.

House, R. (2012). General practice counselling amidst the 'audit culture': History, dynamics and subversion of/in the hypermodern National Health Service. *Psychodynamic Practice*, 18(1), 51–70.

House, R. & Bohart, A. C. (2008). Empirically supported/validated treatments as modernist ideology, II: Alternative perspectives on research and practice. In R. House & D. Loewenthal (eds), *Against and for CBT: Towards a constructive dialogue?* (pp. 202–217). Ross-on-Wye, UK: PCCS Books.

House, R. & Loewenthal, D. (eds) (2008). *Against and for CBT: Towards a constructive dialogue?* Ross-on-Wye, UK: PCCS Books.

House, R. & Totton, N. (eds) (2011a). *Implausible professions: Arguments for pluralism and autonomy in psychotherapy and counselling*, 2nd edn. Ross-on Wye, UK: PCCS Books (orig. 1997).

House, R. & Totton, N. (2011b). Introduction. In R. House & N. Totton (eds), *Implausible professions: Arguments for pluralism and autonomy in psychotherapy and counselling* (pp. 9–18). Ross-on-Wye, UK: PCCS Books (orig. 1997).

House, R. Karian, P. & Young, J. (2011). Power, diversity and values-congruent accountability in the psychological therapies: Report on an emerging dialogue. *Psychotherapy and Politics International*, 9(3), 174–87.

Hursh, D. W. (2006). Marketing education: The rise of standardized testing, accountability, competition, and markets in public education. In E. W. Ross and R. Gibson (eds), *Neoliberalism and education reform* (pp. 1–34). Cresskill, NJ: Hampton Press.

Hursh, D. W. (2007). Neoliberalism and the control of students, and learning: The rise of standards, standardization, and accountability. In E. W. Ross & R. Gibson (eds), *Neoliberalism and education reform*. Cresskill, NJ: Hampton Press.

Johnson, E. L. & Sandage, S. J. (1999). A postmodern reconstruction of psychotherapy: Orienteering, religion and the healing of the soul. *Psychotherapy: Theory, Research, Practice, Training*, 36, 1–15.

Kilroy, P., Bailey, R. & Chare, N. (2004). Editorial sounding: Auditing culture. *Parallax*, 31, 10(2), 1–2.

King, L., & Moutsou, C. (eds) (2010). *Rethinking audit cultures: A critical look at evidence-based practice in psychotherapy and beyond*. Ross-on Wye, UK: PCCS Books.

Kuhn, T. S. (1977). *The essential tension: Selected studies in scientific tradition and change*. Chicago, IL: University of Chicago Press.

Kvale, S. (ed.) (1992). *Psychology and postmodernism*. London: Sage.

Large, M. (2010). *Common wealth*. Stroud, UK: Hawthorn Press.

Lees, J. (1997). An approach to counselling in GP surgeries. *Psychodynamic Practice*, 3(1), 33–48.

Levin, D. M. (ed.) (1987). *Pathologies of the modern self: Postmodern studies on narcissism, schizophrenia, and depression.* New York: New York University Press.

Lowe, R. (1999). Between the 'no-longer' and the 'not-yet': Postmodernism as a context for critical therapy work. In I. Parker (ed.), *Deconstructing psychotherapy* (pp. 71–85). London: Sage.

Mace, C., Moorey, S. & Roberts, B. (eds) (2001). *Evidence in the psychological therapies: A critical guide for practitioners.* London: Routledge.

McCarthy J. & Rose, P. (2010). *Values-based health and social care: Beyond evidence-based practice.* London: Sage.

McGilchrist, I. (2012). *The master and his emissary: The divided brain and the making of the western world*, 2nd edn. New Haven, CT: Yale University Press (orig. 2007).

Miller, H. T. (2002). *Postmodern public policy.* Albany, NY: State University of New York Press.

Miller, J.-A. (2007). The era of the man without qualities. *Psychoanalytic Notebooks* (London Society of the New Lacanian School), 16, 7–42.

Mowbray, R. (1995). *The case against psychotherapy registration: A conservation issue for the human potential movement.* London: Trans Marginal Press; downloadable as a pdf file free of charge at: www.transmarginalpress.co.uk.

Nadler, G., Hibino, S. & Farrell, J. (1995). *Creative solution finding: The triumph of breakthrough thinking over conventional problem solving.* Rocklin, CA: Prima.

Nolan, J. L. (1998). *The therapeutic state: Justifying government at century's end.* New York: New York University Press.

Noys, B. (2014). *Malign velocities: Accelerationism and capitalism.* Alresford, UK: Zero Books.

Olssen, M. & Peters, M. A. (2005). Neoliberalism, higher education and the knowledge economy: From the free market to knowledge capitalism. *Journal of Education Policy*, 20(3), 313–45.

Parker, I. (ed.) (1999). *Deconstructing psychotherapy.* London: Sage.

Parker, I., Georgaca, E., Harper, D. & McLaughlin, T. (1995). *Deconstructing psychopathology.* London: Sage.

Parker, M. (2002). *Against managerialism: Organization in the age of managerialism.* Cambridge: Polity.

Peck, J. (2012) *Constructions of neoliberal reason.* Oxford: Oxford University Press.

Peters, M. A. (2013). Managerialism and the neoliberal university: Prospects for new forms of 'open management' in higher education. *Contemporary Readings in Law and Social Justice*, 1, 11–26.

Pilgrim, D. (2008). Reading 'happiness': CBT and the Layard thesis. In R. House & D. Loewenthal (eds), *Against and for CBT: Towards a constructive dialogue?* (pp. 256–68). Ross-on-Wye, UK: PCCS Books.

Power, M. (1994a). *The audit explosion.* London: Demos.

Power, M. (1994b). The audit society. In A. Hopwood & P. Miller (eds), *Accounting as social and institutional practice* (pp. 299–316). Cambridge: Cambridge University Press.

Power, M. (1997). *The audit society: Rituals of verification.* Oxford: Oxford University Press.

Power, M. (1998). The audit fixation: Some issues for psychotherapy. In R. Davenhill & M. Patrick (ed.), *Re-thinking clinical audit: The case of psychotherapy services in the NHS* (pp. 23–37). London: Routledge.

Ranson, S. (2003). Public accountability in the age of neoliberal governance. *Journal of Education Policy*, 18(5), 459–80.

Rizq, R. (2014). Perversion, neoliberalism and therapy: The audit culture in mental health services. *Psychoanalysis, Culture and Society*, 19, 209–18.

Rorty, R. (1991). Introduction: Pragmatism and post-Nietzschean philosophy. In R. Rorty (ed.), *Essays of Heidegger and Others* (pp. 1–6). New York: Cambridge University Press.

Rose, T., Loewenthal, D. & Greenwood, D. (2005). Counselling and psychotherapy as a form of learning: Some implications for practice. *British Journal of Guidance and Counselling*, 33(4), 441–56.

Schaef, A. W. (1992). *Beyond therapy, beyond science: A new model for healing the whole person.* New York: HarperCollins.

Schön, D. A. (1983). *The reflective practitioner: How professionals think in action.* New York: Basic Books.

Scott, J. C. (1999). *Seeing like a state: How certain schemes to improve the human condition have failed.* New Haven, CT: Yale University Press.

Secretary of State for Health. (2007). Trust, assurance and safety – The regulation of health professionals in the 21st century. White Paper, February; Cm 7013.

Shore, C. (2010). Audit culture and illiberal governance: Universities and the politics of accountability. In L. King & C. Moutsou (eds), *Rethinking audit cultures: A critical look at evidence-based practice in psychotherapy and beyond* (pp. 11–36). Ross-on Wye, UK: PCCS Books; also in *Anthropological Theory*, 8(3), 2008: 278–98.

Smail, D. (1983). Psychotherapy and psychology. In D. Pilgrim (ed.), *Psychology and psychotherapy: Current trends and issues* (pp. 7–20). London: Routledge and Kegan Paul.

Smail, D. (1987). Psychotherapy and 'change': Some ethical considerations. In S. Fairbairn & G. Fairbairn (eds), *Psychology, ethics and change* (pp. 31–43). London: Routledge and Kegan Paul.

Smail, D. (1996). *How to survive without psychotherapy.* London: Constable.

Steiner, R. (1919/1996). *The threefold social order.* London: New Economy Publications.

Styhre, A. (2014). *Management and neoliberalism: Connecting policies and practices.* London: Routledge.

Tarnas, R. (1991). *The passion of the western mind: Understanding the ideas that have shaped our world view.* New York: Ballantine Books.

Thorpe, C. (2008). Capitalism, audit, and the demise of the humanistic academy. *Workplace*, 15, 103–25.

Totton, N. (2011). Introduction. In R. House & N. Totton (eds), *Implausible professions: Arguments for pluralism and autonomy in psychotherapy and counselling*, 2nd edn. (pp. 1–8). Ross-on Wye, UK: PCCS Books.

Trifonas, P. P. (2004). Auditing education: Deconstruction and the archiving of knowledge as curriculum. *Parallax*, 31, 10(2), 37–49.

Trinder, L. & Reynolds, S. (eds) (2000). *Evidence-based practice: A critical appraisal.* Oxford: Blackwell.

van Deurzen, E. (2009). *Psychotherapy and the quest for happiness.* London: Sage.

van Manen, M. (1986). *The tone of teaching.* Richmond Hill, Ontario: TAB Publishers.

Woodhouse, M. (1996). *Paradigm wars: World views for a new age.* Berkeley, CA: Frog.

Woolfolk, R. L. (2002). The power of negative thinking: Truth, melancholia, and the tragic sense of life. *Journal of Theoretical and Philosophical Psychology*, 22(1), 19–27.

12

CONCLUDING THOUGHTS

John Lees

> It only takes two generations of materialism and disruption of spiritual values and the human being will degenerate, fall into decay, and we will be corrupted in our morality, and in our mental and physical health.
>
> Rudolf Steiner, Karma of Vocation

Introduction

This book has investigated the changes which have been taking place within the therapy profession and within society at large as a result of the increasing influence of managerial thinking in the early years of the twenty-first century in the form of the IAPT scheme. But, whether we are working with IAPT or not, it is a manifestation of a prevailing way of thinking, which, arguably, will gradually affect all of us. The evolution of the new BACP Ethical Framework, which was adopted in 2015, is a case in point. The process illustrates both the dangers facing us and the importance of wakefulness in the present climate. My attention was drawn to this issue by a talk at the Universities Psychotherapy and Counselling Association annual conference towards the end of 2014 after the initial consultation about the proposed changes.[1] The talk referred to the current tendency, within the profession, to look at 'the alleviation of distress without any acknowledgement that any such understanding needs to be embedded within a contextual understanding concerned with meaning' (Musgrave, 2014). It argued that a 'contextual understanding' was embedded throughout the original Ethical Framework but that the proposed changes were 'in some respects more prescriptive' and included 'straightforwardly normative' aspects. In short, the author argued that 'standardization' was embedded in the new proposals (ibid.) – that is to say, his views reflected the concerns expressed in this book. Others also began to express concerns. A petition which accumulated 595 signatures in 4 days was submitted to the BACP by their deadline (Bowes,

2014). Although I have not analysed the process in detail the final document, in my view, is reasonable. So, the episode demonstrates both the dangers of current developments and the possibilities of conscious and aware action.

Concerns about ethics are also raised in Nick Totton's chapter in which he challenges us to think about them from the point of view of the practitioner rather than the bureaucrat. As he says, ethics documents tend to become rules and laws as opposed to rightness:

> we follow ethical principles because we believe them to be right; and belief, in this context, is not something centred on our reason, and certainly not centred on someone else's reason, but something we experience as an embodied sense of 'rightness' about one course of action and 'wrongness' about another one.

The discussion around ethics is just one example of the direction of the thinking in the profession and the need for vigilance. Other far-reaching changes have been introduced into the profession in the early years of the twenty-first century – attempts to bring about regulation, managed care and increased bureaucratization, the introduction of manualization, evidence-based practice and of course IAPT as the pinnacle of some of these principles. The tendency is towards prescriptive, normative and standardized elements as opposed to an appreciation of the context, complexity, unpredictability and meaning-making, which forms the essence of therapy.

These developments are likely to intensify in the future. We are, as noted by Samuels (2014, p. 189), going to experience 'more pressure on us to conform' in the future. Are we equipped, as he points out, to 'resist State pressure for conformity?' The book's response to this challenge has two primary aspects. First, it has examined the nature of the threats to the traditions of therapy practice and the probable consequences of this for the future. Second, in spite of these concerns, it highlights a different way forward for the profession, based on the realities of practice. The contributors remind us of how, during the period in which managed care and evidence-based practice have been growing and developing, there have been other innovatory and hopeful developments, which we need to take into account if we are to build a balanced profession.

The problems of managed care

The book offers many insights into the problems of managed care and how it affects the way in which we think about psychological problems. There are many aspects to this. The contributors consistently comment in a variety of ways on how managed care ignores the social and political context of therapeutic work. In this section, I will look at some of these observations. I will then go on to look at possible future scenarios arising out of this.

Observations

The observations about managed care fall into three main areas: its fundamental nature, its deeper unacknowledged aspects, and its effects.

Managed care is top down in orientation and is based on the technical rational principles of problem solving as opposed to the practical wisdom of practitioner experience (Kinsella, 2007). Its protocols and stepped care principles are based, as Richard House remarks, on a 'narrowly circumscribed, instrumental "technology"' which 'bears little if any relation to the kind of authentic' therapy of many practitioners. It is underpinned by a 'narrowly stultifying materialistic thinking' and an 'ideology of standardization'. It is, as he says, a form of 'statist therapy'. The theme of standardization is also picked up by Stuart Morgan-Ayrs, who points out how this goes against the needs of clients. Indeed, a major flaw in the system is the lack of scope for the creation of new ideas, theories and perspectives – in stark contrast to the twentieth century when new ideas proliferated in the profession.

The rhetoric of IAPT is powerful. It has a tendency, as Jay Watts points out, to promote unrealistic expectations in patients. In addition, Ian Simpson speaks about the 'fantasy of discovering a "perfect", all-encompassing understanding of how we function together', while Rosemary Rizq speaks about the way in which the system is driven by anxiety in the face of an unmanageable level of psychological distress created in society today. As Richard House says 'Western culture is teetering under the weight of unprecedented levels of unacknowledged and unprocessed anxiety'.

The effects of the system are pervasive. First, it leads, as Jay Watts says, to an inability to listen to the insight and experience of grassroots practitioners who are implementing the scheme and facing its day to day realities. It also carries the danger of ignoring the knowledge base of therapy, which has been built up over more than one hundred years. Second, and following on from this, it affects, as Ian Simpson describes, the work of practitioners and well-established organizations leading to the demise of many voluntary and community organizations. In particular, he describes the experience of an organization which was functioning very well, had a strong therapeutic underpinning based on group and organizational dynamics, but was undermined by an economic and political climate which turned it into a traumatized organization. Third, those which survive and participate in the scheme, as John Nuttall says, can lose their work identity as a result of losing sight of the social consequences of their endeavours. Fourth, and perhaps most importantly, it affects our dignity as human beings. As Jay Watts points out, the self becomes 'a project which can be moulded and chipped away at so as to become attractive to the market' and, even worse, 'people question their own mental health and doubt their capacity to cope' as illustrated in an extremely powerful, and disturbing, case vignette in her chapter. Finally, and in summary, there is a political aspect to the developments. Del Loewenthal speaks about therapy as social control, Nick Totton speaks about Big Brother, and Richard House speaks about the dangers of beginning to think like the State.

The future

I am concerned about the long-term effects of this. In the words of the Buddha 'We are shaped by our thoughts; we become what we think'. So, if we treat people in a standardized way, if we base our principles on fantasy, deny the existence of the reality of anxiety and exercise social control, then people will become standardized, will be unable to connect with reality, unable to process their anxiety and, in effect, will become socially controlled. In other words, we will progressively lose our humanity. But this has been going on for some time as a result of the way governments 'use' people. It is thus not surprising that levels of violence to each other, both physical and psychological, without remorse, became endemic in the twentieth century. In the words of the epigraph to this chapter it has led to a 'disruption of spiritual values' and, as a result of this, the human being has begun to 'degenerate, fall into decay' and we have become 'corrupted in our morality, and in our mental and physical health', words which were written in the middle of the mindless carnage of World War I. But that was one hundred years ago and just the beginning. I am now concerned about the next hundred years.

Some ominous signs about the future are flagged up in this book. Nick Totton refers to a future where CCTV surveillance may be installed in the therapy room. Stuart Morgan-Ayrs refers to George Orwell's *1984*, and Nick Totton implies the same thing in his comment about Big Brother and, as indicated in *1984*, history becomes re-written. As Jay Watts has said, there are already 'discursive moves to rubbish what was before'. As a consequence, over one hundred years of the development of the therapy profession may be forgotten, as attempts are made to develop a one-sided and uni-dimensional 'psychological therapy' professional culture. The book is a reminder that there is a rich and extensive therapy profession which has developed since the end of the nineteenth century and which, as John Nuttall illustrates, is still being delivered within a vibrant and socially conscious third sector and of course private practice. The profession did not begin with the advent of IAPT in 2006.

I have wondered whether, if the present trend is allowed to continue unabated, we will be facing, by 2030, a profession in which practitioners are surplus to needs in therapy. As the links between human intelligence and non-biological intelligence increase, the present usage of technology, such as computerized cognitive-behavioural therapy (CBT) will be extended. Therapy will then be conducted by computers rather than by living human beings. Furthermore, it may become shaped by scientific inventions. I spoke to one scientist who mentioned, quite seriously, that he was thinking about a hat for depression. A hat for depression with fine electrodes fitted to the brain is not beyond the imagination. If the speed of technological invention keeps up its present pace – and there is every reason to think that it will speed up even more – many things will be possible that we can hardly imagine (robotic therapists, interactive virtual therapists using holograms, widespread computerized treatment, and so on).

Technological advancement is not, of course, a bad thing. I am a realist and not a Luddite. But it needs to be used responsibly. And this is where the problem lies. There are too many human beings who use technology for their own ends – usually to make money or to have power over others. The control of the profession, to use George Orwell's terms, will lie with the Inner Party – academic quantitative researchers. This will then be supported by the Outer Party and the Ministry of Truth, which controls public opinion (similar to Nick Totton's prediction about the 'Thought Police') and, of course, history will be re-written. Finally, there will be those practitioners, like myself, whom we can call the proles, who will base our work on the reality of direct lived experience.

These thoughts reflect the view, expressed at the end of the previous section, and implied in many chapters in one form or another, that 'our behaviour and attitudes are influenced and indeed moulded by the discourses and narratives which we encounter'. So there is a danger that we will begin to think in this way without becoming aware of it. We will thereby unconsciously succumb to a creeping conformity to what society's elites want us to think (or not think).

Having said that, I want to emphasize that the book is not just about critiquing managed care but about cultivating creative leading edge therapy practice. So I will look at this aspect of the book in the next section.

Expertise, innovation and hope

The profession, which I would date to the publication of *Studies in Hysteria* by Breuer and Freud in 1895, has built up a wealth of expertise and insight into dealing with psychological problems, and this has not diminished. In the period during which managed care has developed in the UK since the 1980s, there have been many new insights. Innovation has continued. So, in this section, I will look at how expertise, innovation and hope have been expressed in the book. I will show how the book highlights possibilities inherent in reality-based and transformative counselling and psychotherapy as it has developed over the years. In so doing it will be apparent that there are many synergies and overlaps between the different chapters which show how the book could contribute to forming a basis for a coherent alternative to managed care and evidence-based practice.

Expertise

All of the contributors demonstrate their expertise in 'diagnosing' the limitations and problems of managed care and thereby, to use the words of Rosemary Rizq, identifying why government policies fail so often. They also demonstrate, based on many years' experience, how we can approach therapeutic activity and the tensions in professional life in a way which takes into account the whole human being and the reality of human suffering. Stuart Morgan-Ayrs speaks about the need for therapy to incorporate the exploration of 'truth, melancholia and tragedy' of the human condition. Ian Simpson speaks about looking at the whole human being in a way which incorporates the inevitability of anxiety as opposed to brushing it aside and suppressing it as a result of promulgating systems and protocols.

He describes a 'bottom up' approach to therapy which is built on 'staff and patient relational dynamics' and shows how this, rather than a top-down approach, can manage anxiety using our human capacity for containment: 'A supportive setting . . . that is safe enough for our patients to begin to trust and take risks as the treatment or therapeutic process . . . goes through the different phases of illness and wellness'. At the end of the day, as pointed out by Nick Totton, we are helping clients to address the 'tragic irony' of freeing people from 'their own internal surveillance, the inner critic installed in childhood', or what he calls the 'Life Police'.

Innovation

The book examines a range of innovations which have developed in the profession over the years. These broadly fall into four interlinked areas – therapy as diversity, therapy as microcosm and complexity, the attitude of the practitioner and innovations in therapy research.

As regards diversity, I will begin with Del Loewenthal's notion of therapy as cultural practice. This suggests that practice is a diverse activity: a point which is also taken up by Nick Totton, who notes that 'no two therapies – let alone two therapists – are the same', and Richard House, who speaks about the uniqueness of each therapeutic encounter. In effect, research into practice can only realistically be undertaken with samples of one. This suggests the notion of the 'science of the unique' – a term used by a nursing academic to describe the nature of the research undertaken by practitioners in which 'no two settings of clinical encounters are ever the same' (Rolfe, 2006, p. 39). When we undertake clinical practice we are in a continuous process of 'generating *informal* theories', testing them, modifying practice, reformulating theories and so on 'in a reflexive spiral' (p. 40). The science of the unique has important consequences for how we relate to the generalized systems of managed care and evidence-based practice: 'rather than practice being informed by science . . . . practice should re-formulate itself as science' (p. 40).

Del's chapter also points to the notion of therapy as a complex microcosm of therapeutic activity. He emphasizes that therapy should be able to explore anything that seems appropriate and not just the agendas set up by managed care. This might include subversive thoughts, uncomfortable thoughts, fantasies and dreams and looking at meanings within the specific context in which the work takes place – what Richard House refers to as a 'counter-cultural space' in which the 'unthinkable can begin to be thought'. Nick Totton adds to this with the notion of the therapeutic encounter as a complex interaction:

> the therapy room is in fact a place where not just individuals but whole networks encounter each other represented by the therapist and the client – networks that extend through time and space via relationships of family, of work, of friendship and identification.

Ian Simpson's chapter and my own look at complexity from the point of view of the bio–psycho–social nature of therapy (I also add a spiritual aspect) and discuss the complexity of the relational turn in therapy. This brings in the issue of holism, also discussed by Richard House, who refers to therapy as a 'post-modern cosmology, where we can never totally predict or control the phenomena being studied' and in which we need to 'embrace ambiguity, not-knowing the intuitive and the mysterious'. The principle of complexity and depth is carried even further if we take into account the notion of health as well as illness – the principle of salutogenesis, which is mentioned by William Bento, Richard House and me. As William Bento says, therapy is not just about treating symptoms but also about finding 'opportunities for strengthening and guiding the person to find healthy ways of living'.

As regards the attitude of the practitioner, Nick Totton challenges us to think of therapy as 'deliberate risk taking'. He speaks of this as an 'ethical requirement' inasmuch as it is 'the only way to mitigate the dangers of unconscious risk taking'. He also encourages a mood of 'relaxed spontaneity' where we do not attempt to follow a programme but allow responses to arise in us. In fact, in my chapter I reflect on moments when I fail to do this as a result of my internalized managed care system. The primacy of spontaneity is also taken up by other contributors. Del Loewenthal speaks about the 'delusion' of theory and sees therapy, instead, as a cultural practice and Richard House refers to the 'spontaneous co-creation of the human encounter' as the core dimension of therapeutic practice.

While on the issue of attitude I also wanted to say that the chapter by Jay Watts highlighted the need for a particular attitude to the changes in the profession. Although speaking mainly about the limitations of IAPT (including an astute analysis of CBT as practised in IAPT) her chapter pointed to the need to fructify the limitations of IAPT with transformational approaches to practice. Rather than inculcating clients with a sense of 'who they are and how, from now on, they must act' based on moulding and chipping away at them 'so as to become attractive to the market' it evoked for me the antidote to this; namely to work towards liberating our clients to be themselves. Indeed this is an underlying sentiment that pervades all of the chapters in the book.

Rosemary Rizq's chapter and mine speak about innovation in clinical research and demonstrate how creative research methods can be used to illuminate therapy practice. Rosemary uses autoethnography to investigate a clinical vignette while I use transformational research to investigate my actions in response to developments in the profession in recent years. Such methodologies focus on the particular but, in so doing, as she says, help us to 'understand something of the "universal"'. It is about realities rather than abstractions and fantasy policies. As Tennessee Williams is reputed to have said: 'If I try to make a universal character, it becomes boring. It doesn't exist. If I make the character specific and concrete, it becomes universal'. The unique and micro element of research into practice enables us, as she says, to come to a 'richer, more informative understanding of organizational life' – or, indeed, any aspect of human experience.

Hope

The systems we are facing in the world today are not monolithic and cast in stone forever. The beginning of the twenty-first century – and the developments in therapy which are taking place at this moment in time – is just that; a moment in time. It is therefore important to be able to see beyond the present situation and not be overwhelmed with despair – to take into account the constantly evolving and changing nature of professional life as a result of developing 'an evolutionary kind of thinking', which is equipped to observe 'the growing, changing being of Man' (Welburn, 2004, p. 48). We can then reflect on whether the problem is outside us in the world or within us owing to the way in which we have internalized the systems – the notion of 'Foucauldian subjectification', as discussed by Stuart Morgan-Ayrs.

Stuart Morgan-Ayrs also shows how, in spite of attempts to introduce statutory registration in the profession, there is still a diversity of possibilities in registration systems as a result, for instance, of the introduction of voluntary registration. As he says, it is important for practitioners to co-operate with such systems in order to make them work so as to make statutory registration redundant. There is also an alternative to managed care and, in this chapter, I have been attempting to show how the book opens up this possibility. To develop this further we need to build on the core values of therapy, which Richard House refers to in detail. Both John Nuttall and I also take up the issue of values. In our chapters, we look at the clash of values between IAPT and the values underpinning this book. John Nuttall, basing his view on his experience of IAPT, refers to the fact that, as it currently operates, there is some flexibility in the system, which allows for the utilization of integrative, psychodynamic and humanistic approaches. In fact three of the practitioners writing in this book – Rosemary Rizq, Jay Watts and John Nuttall – have worked with IAPT even though they have not been trained in the evidence-based culture which it supports. In spite of the pressures to limit IAPT to evidence-based therapies and to impose systems and protocols on practitioners, the reality, at a grassroots level, is not always so rigid and inflexible and never can be as long as human beings, as opposed to systems, are able to maintain their integrity and continue to be the driving force in the development of the therapy profession.

Conclusion

The book has had the primary aim of awakening practitioners to what is actually going on around them in the therapy profession as a result of the pervasive influence of the dominant discourse of managed care and evidence-based practice. It has also discussed how the marginalized relational discourse is usually ignored by policy makers. There is little dialogue, communication or exchange of ideas between the two; only a tendency to engage in polemic in relation to each other. The book began with concerns about the systems that are dominant in therapy and healthcare today (Mainly Context), then examined managed care (Mainly IAPT) and finally looked at some innovative ideas which have been developed in our profession over the years including the years when managed care has been dominant (Mainly Practice). Yet this is just a beginning. There is still much more to be done. Therapy is still the leading edge. I agree with Richard House that 'psychological therapies should surely be at the forefront' of developments in society today. The views expressed in the book bring the challenges facing the profession today into sharp relief, as we routinely do with the problems of our clients. But, having done this, we also have the tools to solve the problem, as we do in our clinical work.

Note

1 'Psychotherapy and counselling: from cottage industry to factory production – can we survive, do we want to?' Universities Psychotherapy and Counselling Association (UPCA) conference, the University of Roehampton, 22 November 2014.

References

Bowes, M. (2014). Stop BACP squeeze on counselling professions. Retrieved in August 2015 from: www.thepetitionsite.com/en-gb/332/443/030/stop-bacp-squeeze-on-the-counselling-professions/#sign.

Kinsella, E. A. (2007). Technical rationality in Schön's reflective practice: Dichotomous or non-dualistic epistemological position. *Nursing Philosophy, 8*, 102–13.

Musgrave, A. (2014). The emergence of 'State-endorsed therapy'. . . . ? Retrieved in February 2015 from: https://arthurmusgrave.wordpress.com/.

Rolfe, G. (2006). Nursing practice and the science of the unique. *Nursing Science Quarterly, 19*(1), 39–43.

Samuels, A. (2014). Shadows of the therapy relationship. In D. Loewenthal & A. Samuels (Eds.), *Relational psychotherapy, psychoanalysis and counselling* (pp. 184–92). London: Routledge.

Welburn, A. (2004). *Rudolf Steiner's philosophy*. Edinburgh, UK: Floris Books.

INDEX

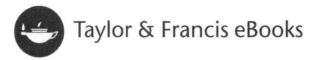 Taylor & Francis eBooks

Helping you to choose the right eBooks for your Library

Add Routledge titles to your library's digital collection today. Taylor and Francis ebooks contains over 50,000 titles in the Humanities, Social Sciences, Behavioural Sciences, Built Environment and Law.

Choose from a range of subject packages or create your own!

Benefits for you

» Free MARC records
» COUNTER-compliant usage statistics
» Flexible purchase and pricing options
» All titles DRM-free.

REQUEST YOUR **FREE** INSTITUTIONAL TRIAL TODAY

Free Trials Available
We offer free trials to qualifying academic, corporate and government customers.

Benefits for your user

» Off-site, anytime access via Athens or referring URL
» Print or copy pages or chapters
» Full content search
» Bookmark, highlight and annotate text
» Access to thousands of pages of quality research at the click of a button.

eCollections – Choose from over 30 subject eCollections, including:

Archaeology	Language Learning
Architecture	Law
Asian Studies	Literature
Business & Management	Media & Communication
Classical Studies	Middle East Studies
Construction	Music
Creative & Media Arts	Philosophy
Criminology & Criminal Justice	Planning
Economics	Politics
Education	Psychology & Mental Health
Energy	Religion
Engineering	Security
English Language & Linguistics	Social Work
Environment & Sustainability	Sociology
Geography	Sport
Health Studies	Theatre & Performance
History	Tourism, Hospitality & Events

For more information, pricing enquiries or to order a free trial, please contact your local sales team: www.tandfebooks.com/page/sales

 Routledge
Taylor & Francis Group

The home of Routledge books

www.tandfebooks.com